THE TURKISH LETTERS OF
OGIER GHISELIN DE BUSBECQ

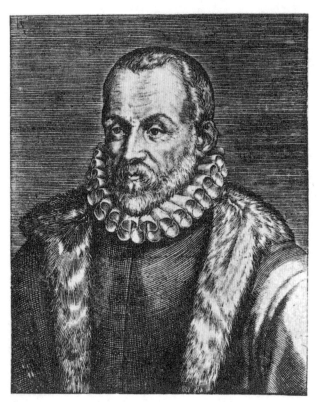

OGIER GHISELIN DE BUSBECQ

THE

TURKISH LETTERS

OF

OGIER GHISELIN DE BUSBECQ

Imperial Ambassador at Constantinople

1554-1562

TRANSLATED FROM THE LATIN
OF THE ELZEVIR EDITION
OF 1633

BY

EDWARD SEYMOUR FORSTER

With a Foreword by Karl A. Roider

LOUISIANA STATE UNIVERSITY PRESS
BATON ROUGE

LIBRARY OF CONGRESS CATALOGING-IN-PUBLICATION DATA

Busbecq, Ogier Ghislain de, 1522–1592.
    [Legationis Turcicae epistolae quatuor. English]
    The Turkish letters of Ogier Ghiselin de Busbecq, imperial
ambassador at Constantinople, 1554-1562 : translated from the Latin of
the Elzevir edition of 1663 / [translated and with an introd. by] Edward
Seymour Forster ; with a foreword by Karl A. Roider.
        p. cm.
    Originally published: Oxford : Clarendon Press, 1927.
    ISBN 978-0-8071-3071-1 (pbk. : alk. paper)
    1. Turkey—Description and travel—Early works to 1800.
    I. Forster, E. S. (Edward Seymour), 1879-1950. II. Title.
    DR423.B8 2005
    956.1'0152—dc22

                                                    2004025536

TO

H. A. O.

IN MEMORY OF A

TOUR IN THE NEAR EAST

LIST OF ILLUSTRATIONS

FOREWORD

THE *Turkish Letters* of Ogier Ghiselin de Busbecq represent the finest contemporary account published in the West of the Ottoman Empire in the latter part of the reign of its most glorious sultan, Suleiman the Magnificent. Interest in the history of the Ottoman Empire has enjoyed a resurgence in recent years because of the troubles in its former provinces such as Bosnia and Kosovo in Europe and Iraq and Israel/Palestine in the Middle East. Traditionally, Western historians have put forth the view that the Ottoman Empire, especially in its later years, was an oppressive, corrupt, overbearing state that treated its subjects— Muslim, Christian, and Jew—with contempt. As the complexities of and difficulties in governing its former lands have become increasingly evident to the modern world, historians have come to appreciate the more tolerant, effective side of Ottoman rule and have argued that perhaps the Empire was not the obscurantist state earlier historians had portrayed it as.

To some extent these revisionist views have contributed to the modern debate about Orientalism, to which Busbecq's *Letters* offer significant insights. Whereas many nineteenth- and twentieth-century Western travelers and scholars viewed the Ottoman Empire and its legacy as backward, impoverished, irrational, sensual, and anti-modern, Busbecq, in a much earlier time, spoke of the Empire's willingness to adapt, to learn, and to lead. "No nation has shown less reluctance to adopt the useful inventions of others," he wrote. "For example, they have appropriated to their own use large and small cannons and many others of our discoveries" (135).

In keeping with his underlying respect for Ottoman politics and culture, Busbecq belongs to that group of observers of Eastern ways who believed that the East had much to teach the West. In one way this perspective was personal, for Busbecq was the natural son of George Ghiselin II, Seigneur de Busbecq, born in 1522 and legitimatized by Holy Roman Emperor Charles V in 1549. Since he was conscious of the stigma of his own illegitimate birth and understood that he could overcome it only by his ability and skill, Busbecq displayed an understandable affinity for what he perceived as a society and political system that prized talent over birth. "Among the Turks, dignities, offices, and administrative posts are the rewards of ability and merit; those who are dishonest, lazy, and slothful never attain to distinction, but remain in obscurity and contempt. . . . Our [Christian Europe's] method is different; there is no room for merit, everything depends on birth" (60). Though Bus-

becq exaggerated the openness of Ottoman politics, there were considerably more opportunities
for men of ability to rise in that system than there
were in any European country.

Busbecq likewise admired the discipline, moderation, and order of the Empire, especially among
its soldiers, and believed that the West had better
learn from the Turks or face ruin at their hands:
"On their side are the resources of a mighty empire, strength unimpaired, experience and practice
in fighting, a veteran soldiery, habituation to victory, endurance of toil, unity, order, discipline, frugality, and watchfulness. On our side is public
poverty, private luxury, impaired strength, broken
spirit, lack of endurance and training; . . . licence,
recklessness, drunkenness, and debauchery . . . ."
If there is war, Busbecq wondered, "Can we doubt
what the result will be?" (112).

Busbecq left on his first mission to the Ottoman
Empire in late 1554 at the age of thirty-two in the
service of Ferdinand of Habsburg, King of the Romans, King of Bohemia and Hungary (1526-64),
and later Holy Roman Emperor (1556-64). Busbecq's only prior experience as a diplomat had been
as witness to the wedding of Philip of Spain and
Mary of England in Winchester Cathedral earlier
that year. His first Turkish letter, addressed to another Habsburg diplomat, Nicholas Michault, and

dated September 1, 1555, resulted from this first mission, which lasted less than a year. The second letter, dated July 14, 1556, marked his return to Constantinople, and the last two letters date from during and after his long embassy that ended in 1562. Although Busbecq told his friend Michault that these letters were not for publication, in fact Busbecq composed the final drafts between 1580 and 1589, two decades after his mission, from notes he took during his time in the Ottoman Empire, precisely for publication. His first letter appeared in print in the original Latin in Antwerp in 1581, and the first edition of all four letters appeared in Paris in 1589, prior to his death in 1592. Over the course of the centuries many other editions appeared, and the *Letters* were translated into a number of European languages.

In the political sphere, perhaps Busbecq's great contribution is his nuanced portrayal of Suleiman (Busbecq's "Soleiman") the Magnificent and his entourage in the latter years of the great Sultan's reign. Busbecq had his first audience with the Sultan not in the capital city of Constantinople but in the interior of Anatolia, where Suleiman was with his army, engaged in peace negotiations with the Persians. Busbecq's portrayal is one of the Sultan in his later years, and it describes particularly the aging Sultan's relationships with his wife and his sons, which were of great importance in the Ottoman Empire at that time as potential successors vied for power. Each sultan who reached the throne had the right to murder any possible rivals, including his brothers. Because of this custom, as a sultan aged there was considerable and urgent jockeying for the succession among his sons, their mothers, ministers, eunuchs of the palace, and the Janissaries, the elite Ottoman infantrymen who formed a kind of palace guard. In the Ottoman Empire the succession was literally a life-or-death matter, for not only would the sons who failed to secure the throne be killed but neither would their supporters escape retribution.

Busbecq in his letters wrote of three sons who were possible successors: Selim, the Sultan's choice; Mustafa, the choice of the Janissaries; and Bayezid, younger brother of Selim and the choice of their mother. Given Busbecq's warnings about the prospect of future wars between the Ottoman Empire and Western Europe, he was probably not unhappy to report the demise of the two talented sons, Mustafa and Bayezid, in favor of the less promising one, Selim, who succeeded his father and earned the moniker "the Sot." He even described Selim in his second letter as a man "naturally gluttonous and slothful," who would therefore hold a "promise of peace" (165). Although he

used that phrase to describe relations between the
Ottomans and the Persians, he undoubtedly believed that Selim would be interested in peace with
the West as well. Perhaps when Busbecq composed
these letters from his notes, he was reflecting on
the significant ebb of the Ottoman threat between
1562 and the 1580s. The ineffectual Selim did succeed in 1566, was himself dead by 1574, and was in
turn succeeded by his equally weak son Murad III.
Whether or not Busbecq sensed it as early as the
1580s, the low quality of the post-Suleiman sultans
marked the beginnings of Ottoman decline.

Politics was by no means the only interest Busbecq revealed in his letters. He was an avid plant
collector, animal observer, gatherer of antiquities,
and numismatist. He is often credited with bringing a number of plants to Western Europe for the
first time, notably the tulip and the lilac. Though
there is some doubt about his introduction of the
tulip, most scholars have no hesitation in crediting
him with the lilac. His pursuit of antiquities generated a wealth of knowledge for Western Europe
about classical Greece and Rome. He gathered, by
his own calculation, 240 classical manuscripts,
some of which scholars credit as real finds, especially a manuscript of Dioscurides, the Greek
physician whose work was the cornerstone of medical herbal therapeutic knowledge for centuries. To

this day this manuscript is regarded as a masterpiece of book art of the classical world. Busbecq donated his treasures to the imperial library in Vienna, and they became the foundation of the classical collection of that distinguished institution. Philologists also credit him with making a significant discovery, described in the fourth letter, of the presence of Goths in the Crimean Peninsula, a remnant of the original German tribes that migrated into the Roman Empire in the first centuries after Christ.

Busbecq's *Letters* represent considerable insights into the Ottoman governmental system at its best, the practice of diplomacy in the sixteenth century, the nature of the Muslim life and practice as interpreted by a Westerner, the world of antiquities and antiquities-gathering, and the everyday culture of many different peoples from long ago. Busbecq was a remarkable observer of his world, and his *Letters* help us appreciate both that world and Busbecq himself as a humanist of the first order.

The translator and introducer of this book, Edward Seymour Forster (1879–1950), was the son of Elizabeth Humphreys Forster and Michael Seymour Forster, the latter the headmaster of Oswestry Grammar School in Oswestry, an old market town in Shropshire near the English-Welsh border. Edward Seymour Forster became a lecturer in classics at the University of Sheffield in 1905, practically upon his graduation from Oriel College, Oxford University. An eminent classical scholar and translator, he remained at Sheffield throughout his academic career, climbing to the rank of professor and retiring in 1945.

Forster was one of the stable of translators for one of the great translation and scholarship projects of the twentieth century, the Loeb Classical Library. James Loeb, who made his fortune from the banking firm of Kuhn, Loeb, and Company, of which his father was a founder, created the Loeb Classical Library with two goals in mind: to make the work of classical authors accessible to a wide reading public untrained in classical languages and to provide a venue to showcase the very best in Anglo-American scholarship. The first twenty publications appeared in 1912, and, even during the First World War, fifty-four new volumes were published. Forster provided translations for a number of Aristotle's works, as well as Florus's *Epitome of Roman History* and Isaeus's *Isaeus.*

In some striking ways Forster and Busbecq had similar experiences. Busbecq was educated in the classics, and his four or five years in the Ottoman Empire marked his introduction to a world outside Western Europe. He was fascinated by antiquities, but he was also intrigued by the contempo-

rary scene in the foreign culture in which he lived
and worked. Forster, a professor of classics, saw the
new Near East as a soldier with the British army
in the Salonica and Black Sea theaters during the
First World War, fighting in a great East/West
conflict that in some ways Busbecq foresaw 350
years earlier. Busbecq was intrigued by the Ottoman Near East of the mid-sixteenth century, and
Forster was intrigued by the increasingly modern
Near East of the early twentieth. As Busbecq
wrote letters of his impressions of what he saw,
Forster, notwithstanding his reputation as a translator of Greek classics, brought the Ottomans and
the land they ruled to the West by publishing Busbecq's *Turkish Letters* and later by writing *A Short
History of Modern Greece* (1946), which was updated
by others following his death in 1950.

As he says in his introduction, Forster came
across a 1633 Latin edition of Busbecq's letters and
was intrigued by their content. He read them first
for entertainment while riding trains and then used
them as illustrative material in some of his lectures.
Because they generated interest among his students, he decided to bring forth a translation with
an introduction that is included in the Louisiana
State University Press edition. Forster notes that,
before his translation, Busbecq's letters had appeared twice before in English, once in 1694 and,

FOREWORD

as part of a larger collection of Busbecq's work, in 1881. Forster's translation is a fluid one, which makes for easy and entertaining reading.

—*Karl A. Roider*

PREFATORY NOTE

THE present translation of the *Turkish Letters* of Busbecq owes its origin to the fact that many years ago a copy of the little Elzevir edition of 1633 came by chance into my possession shortly after a visit to Constantinople. Being a convenient book for the pocket, it served to while away many tedious hours of railway travel, and eventually provided material for a lecture. As the subject matter of the book and the personality of its author aroused some interest, it seemed that it might be worth while to undertake a translation which could be published in a handy form and make the *Letters* accessible to a larger public.

I find that the *Turkish Letters* have already twice appeared in English; first, in an anonymous version, published in London in 1694 (this work is only known to me from bibliographies); secondly, in an elaborate treatise, *The Life and Letters of Ogier Ghiselin de Busbecq*, by C. T. Forster and F. H. B. Daniell in two volumes (London: Kegan, Paul & Co., 1881). The latter work deals with the whole of Busbecq's career, and includes his later correspondence from France with Maximilian and Rudolph; it contains valuable historical notes and appendices, and is indispensable to the historical student who wishes to study Busbecq's career as a whole.

The present translation has the less ambitious aim of presenting only one aspect of Busbecq to the general reader, as the writer of a series of delightful letters which give a unique picture of Turkey in the sixteenth century, and deserve a place by the side of Lady Mary Wortley Montagu's eighteenth-century series of letters and Kinglake's *Eothen*.

In order to bring the work within a reasonable compass, uninteresting matter has been sometimes omitted. Such omissions are always indicated in the text. Brief notes explanatory of the less obvious allusions have been added. The details of Busbecq's life given in the introduction have been mainly derived from the Latin life prefixed to the Elzevir edition.

Those who would know more of Busbecq's later career as an ambassador are referred to the work of Forster and Daniell mentioned above. For the history of Turkey, reference may be made to Von Hammer's *Geschichte des Osmanischen Reiches*, Sir Edward Creasy's *History of the Ottoman Turks*, A. de la Jonquière's *Histoire de l'Empire Ottoman*, and Stanley Lane-Poole's *Turkey* in the ' Story of the Nations ' Series.

I have to thank my friend Professor H. A. Ormerod for kindly reading through the translation in proof.

INTRODUCTION

THE name of Busbecq is familiar to the students of history from the numerous references to his work which are to be found in the foot-notes of Gibbon, Motley, Robertson, and other writers. Numerous editions of his *Turkish Letters*, published in the later sixteenth, the seventeenth, and the early eighteenth centuries, testify to their former popularity, but in more recent times they have fallen into comparative neglect in spite of the fact that they contain the best extant description of the Ottoman Empire at the height of its glory, when it was not merely a preoccupation but an actual menace to Europe. The letters are also full of the quaintest lore and the most delightful stories, several of which are quoted in Burton's *Anatomy of Melancholy*. Diplomatist, traveller, linguist, scholar, antiquarian, zoologist, and botanist, Busbecq was one of those many-sided men who seem to touch no department of human knowledge without making valuable contributions to it. He has a special claim to the attention of the learned world in his profound knowledge of the classical authors, his diligent collection of ancient manuscripts, and his interest in antiquities, inscriptions, and coins. He was the first European to penetrate into certain parts

of Asia Minor since their occupation by the
Turks ; he was the first copyist of the most
famous of all Latin historical inscriptions, the
Monumentum Ancyranum ; and he brought back
to Vienna some 240 classical manuscripts and
greatly enriched the imperial collection of coins.
He has other claims to fame in that he was the
first to introduce the lilac and the tulip into
Western Europe, while his preservation of the
Crim-Gothic vocabulary was a unique contribution to the history of language. Last, but not least,
the *Letters* reveal a charming personality, a man
of the world with a strong sense of humour,
a frank and genial observer of human life.

Ogier Ghiselin de Busbecq was the natural
son of George Ghiselin, Seigneur de Busbecq,
and was born in 1522. His birthplace was
Comines, on the right bank of the river Lys in
Western Flanders, and about ten miles south-
east of Ypres, while the village of Busbecq lies
near at hand on the left bank of the same river,
in what is now the French Département du Nord.
In 1540, in accordance with a common practice
of the day, Charles V issued a patent legitimizing
him as a member of the ancient family whose
name he bears and whose history can be traced
back into the twelfth century.

No one who reads the *Letters* can doubt that

Busbecq received an excellent classical education. He first entered as a student at the local University of Louvain, whence, in accordance with the custom of his time, he migrated first to Paris, thence to Venice, where he was a pupil of Johannes Baptista Egnatius, the friend and correspondent of Erasmus, and afterwards to Bologna and Padua. The astonishing knowledge which he acquired of the classical languages and ancient history stood him in good stead when he came to travel in the Near East.

Busbecq's first introduction to public life occurred in 1554, when he was a member of the special embassy sent by the Emperor Ferdinand to England to attend the marriage of Queen Mary and Philip II of Spain in Winchester Cathedral. It is unfortunate that he has left us no account of this mission, which is only casually mentioned in his letters. Immediately after his return to Flanders he received an urgent summons to proceed to Vienna and undertake the important duties of imperial ambassador at Constantinople.

Soleiman the Magnificent had been on the throne of the Ottoman Empire since the year 1520, and was among the most striking personalities of his age. The sixteenth century produced many notable rulers—Charles V,

Francis I, and Elizabeth among them—and of these Soleiman was a worthy compeer. He is perhaps the most distinguished figure in Turkish history, a man endowed by nature with the highest intellectual and moral gifts. His personal courage and military genius, his sense of justice and his chivalrous conduct towards a brave foe, his devotion to his own religion and his tolerance of other faiths, his munificence and generosity won him the devotion of his subjects and the respect of his enemies. His reign saw the greatest extension of the Turkish power ; the descendants of the tribe of Othman, who had made their first appearance in history only three hundred years before, were lords of a mighty empire which stretched from Bagdad to the Atlantic, and from Mecca almost to the walls of Vienna. To give the barest outline of his achievements would be far beyond our scope. Succeeding his father, the cruel and detested Selim, at the age of twenty-six, he signalized his accession by capturing Belgrade, which had successfully resisted the assault of the greatest of his predecessors, Mohamed the Conqueror, and thus opened to Turkey the rich plains of Hungary. In 1522 the capture of Rhodes, after its heroic defence by the Knights of St. John, set the seal on Soleiman's military glory, while his generous treatment of a gallant foe won him the admiration of Europe. In 1526 he led a vast army northward and defeated Louis II at the fatal battle of Mohacs, which made Hungary for nearly 150 years a Turkish province and Buda a Turkish outpost. It was only by a supreme effort that Vienna was saved from a like fate. Three years later Soleiman returned to the attack ; but by this time a foe had arisen in Charles V who was worthy of his steel, and the Sultan contented himself with ravaging the open country, and in 1533 peace was concluded at Constantinople on terms advantageous to Turkey. But hostilities again broke out and continued over a period of several years until in 1547 Charles V and Ferdinand were forced to ask for peace, and a truce of five years was granted. In 1551 Ferdinand rashly broke faith with the Turks by his invasion of Transylvania ; whereupon the Sultan seized Malvezzi, the imperial ambassador, and flung him into prison, where he remained for two years, and from which he emerged practically a dying man.

It was to succeed Malvezzi that Busbecq was dispatched to Constantinople in 1554. His mission was to check by diplomacy the raids of the Turks into Hungary, which was then practically at their mercy, and, above all, to gain time and give the Empire a breathing space to recruit for a fresh effort. Busbecq amply justified the hopes of his master, and was able to effect much by his quick sympathy and his appreciation of the Turkish character, his love of straightforward dealing, his personal courage, and, above all, by his untiring patience.

The four *Turkish Letters*, which give the full story of his mission, were addressed to Nicholas Michault, who had been Busbecq's fellow student in Italy and was afterwards imperial ambassador to the Portuguese court. They were never intended for publication. Though Busbecq is sometimes apologetic about his style, he writes easy flowing Latin, garnished with classical quotations and allusions. His favourites among the ancient authors seem to have been the elder Pliny and Tacitus ; and we may perhaps trace the influence of the latter in the way in which Busbecq sums up a situation in an epigram. For example, in speaking of the then recent conquest of Mexico and Peru, he concludes quite in the Tacitean style with the words *pietas obtenditur, aurum quaeritur*— ' religion is the pretext, the object is gold.'

Busbecq returned from Turkey in the autumn of 1562 with an established reputation as a diplomatist. It was not long before he again

obtained employment. Philip of Spain proposed to Maximilian that a marriage should be
arranged between the Infanta of Spain and one
of Maximilian's sons, but stipulated that the
young Archdukes Rudolph and Ernest should
be sent to Spain to be educated. To Busbecq
was entrusted the task of accompanying them
thither. On his return Maximilian conferred
on him the honour of knighthood, and afterwards appointed him governor to his four
younger sons. But a still more important post
was in store for him. In 1570 the Archduchess
Isabella was married to Charles IX of France,
and Busbecq was sent with her as master of the
household, afterwards returning to Vienna. On
the death of Charles IX he was again sent to
Paris to bring back the widowed queen, and
then from 1574–92 resided in the French capital
to look after her interests and secure the punctual
payment of her dowry. At the same time he
acted as an unofficial observer in Paris, and his
letters to Maximilian and his successor Rudolph
are full of interesting sidelights on French affairs
at a most important period of European history.

During his absence abroad Busbecq's thoughts
must often have turned to his old home on the
Lys. He had had the château of Busbecq re-
paired, and no doubt hoped to pass his last

years there. But fate had ordained otherwise.
In 1592, in his seventy-first year, he obtained
leave of absence from the Emperor and set out
to revisit his home. While journeying through
Normandy, then much disturbed by civil war,
he and his baggage were seized at Cailly by
soldiers from a neighbouring camp, who professed to be acting by orders of the Governor
of Rouen. Busbecq, courageous as ever, vio-
lently protested and claimed the privileges of
an ambassador and refused to believe that
orders had been given to molest him. His
protests had such an effect that the robbers
restored to him his belongings and escorted
him back to Cailly and then made good their
escape. The Governor of Rouen, on being informed, hastened to make his apologies and
promised that the offenders should be brought
to justice ; but Busbecq replied that he preferred to make his peace with heaven rather
than to take vengeance on his aggressors. Knowing that his end was near, he begged that he
might be conveyed to the neighbouring castle
of Maillot near St. Germain, where eleven days
later he breathed his last on 28 October 1592.
He was buried in the church of St. Germain ;
but his heart was enclosed in a leaden casket
and placed in the family tomb at Busbecq.

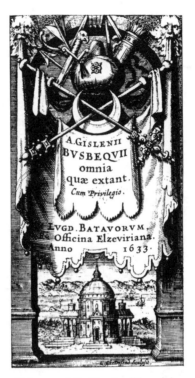

A.GISLENII
BVSBEQVII
omnia
quæ extant.
Cum Privilegio.

LVGD.BATAVORVM,
Officina Elzeviriana.
Anno   1633.

Title-page of the Elzevir edition of the
Turkish Letters, 1633

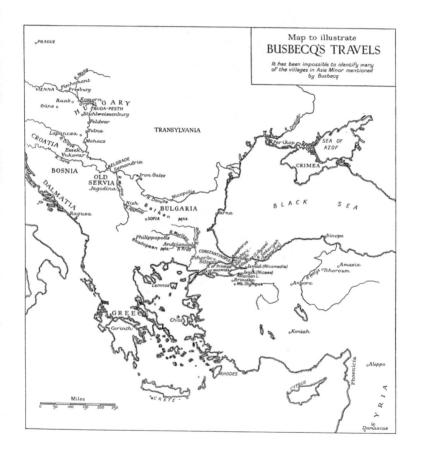

Map to illustrate
BUSBECQ'S TRAVELS

*It has been impossible to identify many
of the villages in Asia Minor mentioned
by Busbecq*

PRAGUE

VIENNA
Fischament
Presburg
R. Waag
Raab
Comorn
Gran
BUDA-PESTH
Güns
Stuhlweissenburg
HUNGARY
Feldvar
Tolna
Lapancsa
Mohacs
Essek
Vukovar
CROATIA
BELGRADE
Semandria
OLD
SERVIA
Jagodina
Iron Gates
BOSNIA
Nish
R. Danube
Nicopolis
Rustova
Balkan Mts.
SOFIA
Mts.
Ragusa
DALMATIA

TRANSYLVANIA

SEA OF
AZOF
Perikop
CRIMEA

BULGARIA
Varna

BLACK   SEA

Philippopolis
Rhodopean Mts.
Andrianople
R. Arda
R. Moritza
CONSTANTINOPLE
Tchorlu
Silivri
Bosphorus
Buyukdere
Pera
Scutari
(Usbunar)
Sinope
Sabanjah
Isnik (Nicaea)
Ismid (Nicomedia)
Ascanian L.
Broussa
Mt. Olympus
R. Halys
Amasia
Tchoroum
Angora
Is. of Prinkipo
S. of MARMORA

Lemnos

GREECE
Chios
Corinth

Koniah

RHODES

CYPRUS

Aleppo

SYRIA

CRETE

Phoenicia

Damascus

Miles
0   50   100   150   200   250

THE FIRST LETTER

Vienna, 1 Sept. 1555 (*n*).

I PROMISED, when I parted from you, that you should
have a full account of my journey to Constantinople.
I am now preparing to fulfil this promise ; nay more,
if I mistake not, I shall discharge the debt with interest,
for to the story of my journey to Constantinople I
intend to add that of my expedition to Amasia, a much
less hackneyed and ordinary undertaking. If you find
that I have met with delightful adventures, you will
partake of my enjoyment ; we are such old friends
that we share in each other's pleasures. If, on the other
hand, as must necessarily happen in a journey of such
length and difficulty, any disagreeable incidents occurred, you must not take them to heart ; they are
past and over, and the greater the annoyance they
caused me at the time the greater is the pleasure which
I take in relating them.

You will remember my return home from attending
the marriage of King Philip and Queen Mary (*n*) in England (where I was in attendance upon Don Pedro Lasso,
whom my most gracious master Ferdinand, King of the
Romans, sent to do honour to the royal pair), and the
summons which I received from Ferdinand to undertake this journey. I was at Lille when his letter reached
me on 3 November, and I only delayed my journey
to turn aside to Busbecq and bid farewell to my father
and my friends, and then hurried through Tournai to
Brussels. There I met Don Pedro himself, and he, as
they say, spurred on the willing horse by showing me
a letter from the King, in which he commanded him to

secure my immediate departure. I therefore hastily took post-horses and hurried to Vienna with all possible speed. It was a trying journey; for I was unaccustomed to this uncomfortable mode of transport, and the season of the year, with its bad weather, muddy roads, and short days, was anything but favourable to travelling. I was obliged to journey far into the night and to hurry in a dangerous manner through the densest darkness over roads which were almost impassable.

On my arrival in Vienna I was introduced by John Van der Aa, one of the Privy Counsellors, into the presence of Ferdinand, who welcomed me with those marks of goodwill which His Majesty always shows towards those of whose loyalty and honesty he has conceived a favourable opinion. He was eloquent of the hopes which he entertained of my mission and of the importance which he attached to my acceptance of the embassy and my immediate departure. He had given an undertaking to the Pasha of Buda that his representative should reach Buda without fail by the beginning of December, and he was anxious not to give the Turks any excuse, by unpunctuality on his part, for not performing the engagements which they had made in reliance on his promise.

Barely twelve days remained—a brief period to prepare for a short journey, all too brief when so long a journey lay before me. Even from this short space several days had to be subtracted that I might pay a visit, by the King's wish and command, to John Maria Malvezzi at Komorn. His Majesty deemed it most important that, since I had no knowledge or experience of Turkish affairs, I should meet Malvezzi and obtain from his lips some information about their customs and character and advice about their previous policy. Malvezzi had been for some years Ferdinand's representative at the court of Soleiman, in fact ever since the Emperor Charles had, for very good reason, made the truce with the Turks which was negotiated by Gerard Velduvic (*n*); for on that occasion he had made an eight years' truce in the name of King Ferdinand as well. Malvezzi had been attached to Velduvic's mission, and on his return Ferdinand had sent him back to Constantinople as his representative.

[Busbecq then tells how Malvezzi had been thrown into prison by the Turks, when Ferdinand annexed Transylvania, and barbarously ill treated, and had eventually been released and had returned to Vienna. He was setting out again for Constantinople when he was taken ill at Komorn.]

The illness caused by Malvezzi's imprisonment broke out again with such violence that, feeling his life to be in danger, he halted and sent a letter to Ferdinand begging him to appoint some one else to his post as ambassador. Ferdinand neither entirely believed nor altogether discredited what Malvezzi said ; but he was inclined to suspect that his desire to withdraw from his post as ambassador was due rather to his recollection of the past and his dread of future hardships than to any serious illness ; yet he thought that it would be hardly seemly to compel one who had done good service to himself and the State to continue a mission which he wished to avoid. The death of Malvezzi a few months later made it quite clear that his illness was neither a pretence nor assumed to suit his own convenience. Thus I was appointed in his place ; but since I was without experience of Turkish politics or manners, the King was of opinion, as I have already said, that it would be well if I visited Malvezzi and were put on my guard by his instruction and advice against Turkish duplicity. So I spent two days with him and learnt, as far as I could in so short a time, the attitude which I ought to adopt and the precautions which I ought to take in my daily intercourse with the Turk.

I then hurriedly returned to Vienna and set myself with all diligence to make the necessary preparations for my journey. But so much was there to do, and so short was the time, that the day appointed for my departure arrived and found me still unready, though the King continued to urge my departure. I spent the whole day from the early hours of the morning arranging my affairs and my baggage, but it was nightfall before my loins were girt up for departure. The gates of Vienna, which are always locked at that hour, were unbarred, and I set out. The Emperor, on his departure that morning for the chase, said that he was sure that before his return in the evening I should be already on my way ; and so I was, though there was only a brief interval between my departure and his return. At 11 p.m. we reached the Hungarian town of Fischament, some ten miles from Vienna ; here we had our supper, for in our hurry we had started without it. Thence we journeyed to Komorn. [Here, to his great annoyance, Busbecq waited in vain for two days for Paul Palinai, who was to accompany him to Buda.] The next day I crossed the Waag and continued my journey towards Gran, the first fortress within the Turkish dominions.

John Pax, the governor of Komorn, had given me
an escort of sixteen of those horsemen whom the Hungarians call hussars, and had ordered them not to quit
me until the Turkish outposts came in sight. The
Governor of Gran had intimated that his men would
meet me half-way. When I had journeyed for three
hours, more or less, over a vast plain, four Turkish
horsemen appeared in the distance. My Hungarians
continued to accompany me, until I ordered them to
retire ; for I was afraid that, if they came too near,
some embarassing quarrel might arise. When the
Turks saw me approaching, they rode up and halted
by my carriage and saluted me. We then proceeded
for some distance conversing together ; for I had a lad
with me who could act as interpreter. I was expecting
no further escort, when, on descending to rather lower
ground, I suddenly found myself surrounded by a troop
of some 150 horsemen. They formed a charming
spectacle to my unaccustomed eyes, with their brightly
painted shields and spears, their jewelled scimitars,
their many-coloured plumes, their turbans of the
purest white, their garments mostly of purple or bluish
green, their splendid horses and fine trappings. Their
officers rode up and welcomed me with courtesy and
congratulated me on my safe arrival, and asked me if
I had had a pleasant journey ; to which question I
made a suitable reply. I was thus escorted to Gran,
which is the name given to a fortress situated on a hill,
below which flows the Danube, and to the neighbouring town lying in the plain, where I put up for the
night. The archbishop of this place, in virtue of his
position of authority and vast wealth, ranks high among
the Hungarian magnates. My accommodation had all

the severity of a camp ; instead of beds, shaggy rugs of rather a rough kind were spread over planks, and there were no mattresses or linen. Thus my followers had their first experience of Turkish luxury ; I had my own bed, which I always carried with me.

Next day the Sanjak-Bey of the place did not cease to urge that I should visit him. This is the title which the Turks give to the commanding officer, whose *sanjak*, that is a gilded bronze ball, is carried as a standard fixed on the point of a spear at the head of a squadron of cavalry. Although I had no letter or recommendation to him, he was so persistent that I had to go and see him. He really only wished to have a look at me, to offer me his courteous salutations, to ask me what my purpose was, to exhort me to promote peace, and to wish me a prosperous journey. On my way to visit him I was surprised by the croaking of frogs in the month of December and in such cold weather ; it was due to the existence of hot sulphur springs which form pools in these regions.

I left Gran for Buda after a breakfast which was destined to serve as my dinner, as there was no halting place until I reached Buda. I set out escorted by the Sanjak-Bey with all his household and the cavalry which he commanded, though I did my best to dissuade him from paying me this honour. The cavalry, when they had passed through the gates, galloped hither and thither and amused themselves by throwing a ball to the ground and then, after urging their horses to full speed, catching it on the point of their spears, and indulging in other similar sports. Among them was a Tartar with long thick hair, who was said to go bare headed in all weathers and in battle, his hair form-

ing sufficient protection against storms or weapons.
The Sanjak-Bey, when he deemed fit, exchanged
farewells with us and returned home, leaving with me
guides for my journey.

As I approached Buda, a few of those whom the
Turks call *chiauses* (cavasses) came to meet me. They
perform the office of attendants and servants, and
carry almost all the orders of the Sultan and the Pashas.
Their profession is considered highly honourable
among their fellow countrymen. I was taken to lodge
at the house of an Hungarian, where more attention
was paid to my baggage and carriages and horses than
to myself. The first concern of the Turks is to secure
the safety of the horses, carriages, and luggage ; for
human beings they think they have taken enough trouble
if they protect them from the severity of the weather.

The Pasha sent a man to visit and salute me. His
name was Tuigon, a name which the Turkish language
also gives to the stork. He begged me to excuse him
if he could not give me an audience for some few days,
as he was confined to his bed by severe illness ; he
promised to attend to me as soon as he recovered.
This circumstance prevented any inconvenience from
the delay of Palinai, and saved the latter from a serious
charge ; for he used all diligence to arrive in time, and
soon made his appearance. The Pasha's illness kept
me a long time at Buda ; it was believed to have been
due to his annoyance at the theft of a large sum of
money which he had secreted somewhere, for he was
commonly reported to be something of a miser. Meanwhile, when he heard that I had with me William
Quacquelben, a man of wide learning and a skilled
physician, he began to try and induce me to send him

to prescribe for him. I willingly agreed, but I came
very near to repenting bitterly my readiness to oblige
him ; for when the Pasha's illness grew daily more
serious, I felt no little fear that, if he went to join
Mahomet in another world, the Turks would allege
that he had been killed by my physician. This would
have involved my worthy friend in danger, while
I myself would have incurred great disgrace as his
accomplice. However, Providence put an end to my
anxiety by restoring the Pasha to health.

At Buda I first came across the Janissaries, which
is the name they give to their footguards. When they
are at their full strength, the Sultan possesses 12,000
of them, scattered throughout his empire, either to
garrison the fortresses against the enemy or to protect
the Christians and Jews from the violence of the populace. There is no village, town, or city of any size in
which there are not some Janissaries to guard the
Christians, Jews, and other helpless folk from the
attacks of malefactors. In the fortress of Buda there
is a perpetual garrison of Janissaries. They wear robes
reaching to their ankles, and on their heads a covering
consisting of the sleeve of a cloak (for this is the account
which they give of its origin), part of which contains
the head, while the rest hangs down behind and flaps
against the neck. On their foreheads rises an oblong
silver cone, gilded and studded with stones of no great
value. These Janissaries generally visited me in pairs,
and, on being admitted to my dining-room, saluted me
with an obeisance and then hastened, almost at a run,
towards me and took hold of my garment or hand as
though they would kiss it, and offered me a bunch of
hyacinths or narcissi. They would then rush back

again to the door at almost the same speed, taking care not to turn their backs upon me ; for this, according to their ideas, is unbecoming. At the door they would take up their stand silent and respectful, their hands crossed on their breast and their eyes fixed upon the ground ; you would think they were monks rather than soldiers. However, on receiving a few little coins, which was all they wanted, they would again make obeisance and utter their thanks in loud tones and depart with every kind of good wish and blessing. Really, if I had not been told that they were Janissaries, I could well have believed that they were a kind of Turkish monk or the members of some kind of sacred association ; yet these were the famous Janissaries who carry such terror wherever they go.

At Buda many Turks were attracted to my table by the lure of my wine, a luxury which they appreciate all the more because they have little opportunity of enjoying it, and which therefore they consume with all the greater avidity whenever they have the chance. I invited them to stay late, but, when I grew tired and rose from the table and retired to my bedroom, they departed, sad at the thought that they were not yet entirely overcome by the wine and could still walk. Presently a slave arrived, who asked on their behalf that I would give them a supply of wine and some silver cups ; they would, they said, spend the night drinking in any odd corner. I gave orders that they should be provided with all the wine that they required and the vessels for which they asked, and they then went on drinking until they all lay stupified on the ground.

The drinking of wine is regarded by the Turks as a serious crime, especially among the older men ; the younger men can commit the sin with greater hope of pardon and excuse. They think, however, that the punishment which they will suffer in a future life will be just as heavy whether they drink much or little, and so, if they taste wine, they drink deep ; the punishment being already deserved, they incur no additional penalty, and they count their drunkenness as all to the good. Such are their ideas about drinking and others which are still more absurd. I once saw an old fellow at Constantinople, who, when he had taken the cup into his hand, began to utter loud cries. When we asked our friends the reason of this, they declared that he wished by these cries to warn his soul to betake itself to some distant corner of his body or else quit it altogether, so that it might not participate in the crime which he was about to commit and might escape pollution by the wine which he was about to swallow.

It would be a long task to describe the city of Buda in detail. It would require a whole book, and a few remarks suitable to a letter must suffice. It lies in a pleasant situation in a very fertile district on sloping ground bordered on one side by vine-clad hills ; on the other side flows the Danube, with Pesth and a view of wide plains beyond. It seems to have been purposely designed to be the capital of Hungary. The city was formerly adorned with the splendid palaces of the Hungarian nobles ; these have now fallen in ruins, or are only prevented from doing so by the liberal use of props. They are inhabited by Turkish soldiers, whose pay only suffices for their daily needs, and does not allow them to mend the roofs or repair the walls of these vast buildings. They care little if the rain comes through or the walls are cracked, as long as they can find a dry place to stable their horses and make their own bed. The upper stories they regard as no concern of theirs, and leave them to be overrun by rats and mice. Moreover, it is characteristic of the Turks to avoid any magnificence in their buildings ; to care for such things is in their opinion a sign of pride, vanity, and self-conceit, as though a man expected immortality and a permanent abode upon this earth. They regard their houses as a traveller regards an inn ; if they are safe from thieves and protected from heat and cold and rain, they require no further luxuries. This is why in the whole of Turkey you would have difficulty in finding even a rich man in possession of a house of any elegance. The common people live in huts and cottages ; but the rich are fond of gardens and baths, and have roomy houses to accommodate their huge establishments, but no well-lighted porticoes or halls worth looking at or anything else magnificent or attractive. The same is practically true of Hungary. Except at Buda, and possibly in Pressburg, you could scarcely find a single city with any at all splendid buildings. This is due in my opinion to the mode of life which the Hungarians have followed through the ages ; devoting themselves to warfare and camp-life and distant campaigns, they have always neglected to put up buildings, and they dwell in cities as though they may shortly have to quit them.

An interesting phenomenon which I observed at Buda is a spring outside the gate on the Constantinople road, the water of which is boiling on the surface, while below you can see fish swimming about, so that you would imagine that they could not be taken out except ready cooked.

At last, on 7 December, we were introduced into the presence of the Pasha, who had recovered from his illness. We tried to mollify him with presents, and then complained of the insolence and misdeeds of the Turkish soldiers and demanded back the places which had been taken from us in violation of the truce and which he had promised in his letter to my sovereign to restore on condition that he sent a representative. [Busbecq describes his unsatisfactory interview with the Pasha.] I effected nothing except the conclusion of a truce pending the arrival of an answer from Soleiman. . . .

Our business at Buda having been thus, as far as was possible, concluded, my companion returned to the King, and I boarded the vessels which were awaiting us on the Danube ; and, when my horses and carriages and attendants had been embarked, we started downstream for Belgrade. This method of travelling was safer and quicker ; for the journey by land to Belgrade would have taken at least twelve days, especially with so much baggage ; and, besides, there would have been danger from the depredations of the *Heydons*. This is the name given by the Hungarians to those who, from being herdsmen, have become soldiers, or rather brigands. There was no danger from them on the river, and the voyage only occupied five days.

The vessel on which I travelled was towed by a rowing-boat with twenty-four oarsmen ; the other boats were propelled each by a pair of longer oars. We never halted by day or night, except for a few hours when the unhappy rowers and sailors refreshed themselves from their incessant toil with food and rest.

The rashness of the Turks seemed to me quite remarkable ; they never hesitated to continue their voyage in
spite of the densest darkness, the absence of any moon
and the violent gales, and they had continually to
encounter danger from the mills and the trunks and
branches of trees which projected from the banks. It
frequently happened that the violence of the wind
caused my boat to come into such violent collision
with the stumps and boughs of trees which overhung
the stream that it seemed to be in imminent danger of
being broken in pieces. In fact, on one occasion part
of the deck was carried away with a loud crash, which
caused me to spring from my bed and admonish the
sailors to be more careful. Their only reply was to
shout out ' *Alaure* ', that is, ' God will protect us ' ;
and all that remained for me to do was to return to
bed and recapture my sleep, if I could. I venture to
prophesy that this method of travelling will some day
prove disastrous.

During our voyage we saw Tolna, a fine Hungarian
town, which deserves mention for the excellence of its
white wine and the courtesy of its inhabitants. We
also noted the fortress of Valpovat (*n*), which stands on
high ground, and other castles and towns, also the
places where the Drave on one side and the Theiss on
the other joins the Danube.

Belgrade itself lies at the confluence of the Save and
Danube. In the extreme angle, as it were, of the promontory between them lies the old town, of ancient
construction and fortified with numerous towers and
a double wall. It is washed on two sides by the said
rivers ; on the side which unites it to the land is a very
strong fortress on higher ground, with many lofty

towers built of squared stones. In front of the city is a large mass of buildings and extensive suburbs inhabited by various races, Turks, Greeks, Jews, Hungarians, Dalmatians, and many others. Indeed it is quite usual throughout the Turkish Empire for the suburbs to be larger than the towns themselves, the towns and suburbs together giving the impression of very large settlements.

This was the first point at which we were offered ancient coins, in which, as you know, I take great delight. William Quacquelben, whose name I have already mentioned, is a devoted and welcome participator in this pursuit of mine. We came across numerous coins, on one side of which was a Roman soldier standing between a bull and a horse, and inscribed 'Taurunum'. It is well known that the legions of Upper Moesia had a stationary camp there.

Twice within the memory of our grandfathers determined attempts were made by the Turks to capture Belgrade, first by Amurath and afterwards by Mahomet, the Conqueror of Constantinople ; but the barbarian attacks failed before the valiant defence of the Hungarians and the Crusaders. At last, in the year 1520, Soleiman at the beginning of his reign arrived before the city with large forces. Finding it deprived of its proper garrison and open to attack owing to the negligence of the young King Louis and the quarrels of the factious Hungarian chiefs, he had little difficulty in reducing it to submission. It is clear that this event threw open the flood-gates and admitted the tide of troubles in which Hungary is now engulfed. Its first approach involved the death of King Louis (n), the capture of Buda, the enslavement of Transylvania, the

overthrow of a flourishing kingdom, and an alarm
among neighbouring nations lest the same fate should
befall them also. These events ought to be a lesson
to the princes of Christendom and make them realize
that, if they wish to be safe, they cannot be too careful
in securing their fortifications and strongholds against
the enemy. The Turkish armies are like mighty rivers
swollen with rain, which, if they can trickle through
at any point in the banks which restrain them, spread
through the breach and cause infinite destruction.
Even so, and with still more terrible results, the Turks,
when once they have burst the barriers which restrain
them, spread far and wide and cause a devastation
which passes all belief.

But it is time to return to Belgrade, so that we may
continue our journey on to Constantinople. When
we had completed the preparations which seemed
necessary for our journey by road, we started for Nish,
leaving on our left Semandria, which lies on the banks
of the Danube and was formerly a stronghold of the
Despots of Serbia. From the higher ground the Turks
showed us the snow-clad mountains of Transylvania
in the far distance, and pointed out the place where
there still remained traces of the piles of Trajan's
Bridge (n).

Having crossed the river which the natives call the
Morava, we put up in the Serbian village of Jagodina,
where we observed the funeral rites of that people,
which differ greatly from our own. The corpse was
laid out in the church with the face exposed ; near it
was placed food, bread and meat, and a cup of wine.
The wife and daughter of the deceased stood near in
their best clothes, the daughter wearing a head-dress

of peacocks' feathers. There was heard wailing and moaning and cries of lamentation ; and they inquired of the dead man what they had done that they deserved to lose him ; in what act or duty or comfort had they failed him ; why did he leave them lonely and wretched ; and so on. The rites were carried out by Greek priests. In the burial-ground were numerous figures carved in wood of stags and roebucks and other such animals mounted on poles or posts. When we asked the meaning of these, we were told that husbands and fathers testified by these monuments to the willing-less and diligence of their wives or daughters in the performance of their domestic duties. On many of the tombs there were also hung locks of hair, which the women and girls had placed there as a sign of mourning for the death of their relatives. We also learnt that it was a local custom that, after the parents had arranged a match between a young man and a girl, the bridegroom should carry off the bride by force ; for it was thought unseemly that a maiden should voluntarily submit to her husband's first embraces.

Not far from Jagodina we encountered a small river which the inhabitants call the Nishava, and we kept it on our immediate right until we reached Nish. A little farther on we saw on its banks, where there remained traces of a Roman road, a small marble column still standing with an inscription in Latin, but so mutilated as to be illegible. Nish is a little town of some consideration, and well populated for that part of the world.

It is time that I should tell you something of the inns which we frequented ; you have probably been long expecting an account of them. At Nish I was lodged in the public inn, or *caravanserai*, as it is called in Turkish. It is the most usual form of lodging in these parts, and consists of a vast building, rather long for its breadth. In the middle is an open space for the baggage, camels, mules, and vehicles. It is usually surrounded completely by a wall some three feet high, adjoining and built into the outer wall of the building. The top of the low wall is flat and about four feet broad, and serves the Turk for bed and dining-table ; on it they also cook their food, for there are fireplaces at intervals built into the outer wall. This space on the top of the wall is the only place which the traveller does not share with the camels, horses, and other animals ; and, even so, these are tethered to the foot of the wall in such a way that their heads and necks project right over it, and they stand there like attendants, while their masters warm themselves and even dine, and at times take bread or fruit or other food from their hands. On this wall also the Turks make their beds, first unfolding a rug, which they generally carry attached to their horse-cloths, and laying a cloak on the top of it. A saddle serves as a pillow, and they wrap themselves up at night in the long robes reaching to their ankles and lined with fur, which they wear in the daytime. Thus they have none of the usual blandishments wherewith to court sleep.

These inns provide no privacy ; everything must be done in public, and the darkness of night alone shields one from the sight of all. This kind of inn inspired me with particular disgust ; for the Turks kept their gaze fixed upon us in astonishment at our habits and customs. I always, therefore, tried to find accommodation beneath the roof of some unhappy Christian ; but their hovels are so small that very often there is no room to place a bed ; so I often slept in a tent or in my carriage.

I sometimes lodged in a Turkish khan. These are most spacious and quite imposing buildings with separate bedchambers. No one is refused admittance, whether Christian or Jew, rich or poor ; the door is open to all alike. They are used by Pashas and Sanjak-Beys when they travel. I was always given as hospitable a reception as if it were a royal palace. It is customary to offer food to all who lodge there ; and so, when dinner-time arrived, an attendant used to present himself with an enormous wooden tray as large as a table, in the middle of which was a dish of barley-porridge with a piece of meat in it. Round the dish were rolls of bread and sometimes a piece of honeycomb. . . .

Sometimes, if I could find no quarters in a house, I put up in a shed. I used to look out for a large, roomy shed, one half of which contained a fireplace and chimney, while the other was intended for the sheep and cattle ; for it is the usual arrangement for the herd or flock and the shepherd to be housed under the same roof. The part where the fireplace stood I used to screen off with the canvas of my tent, and setting up my table and bed by the fire I lived as happy as the King of Persia. My attendants reclined in the other part of the shed on an abundance of clean straw, or fell asleep in the garden or field near the fire on which our meal had been cooked. This fire enabled them to withstand the cold at night, and they were as careful not to let it go out as the Vestal Virgins at Rome in the olden days.

It will perhaps occur to you to ask how I consoled my followers for such bad lodging ; for you will surmise, and quite rightly, that wine, the usual remedy for uncomfortable nights, is not too plentiful in the middle of Turkey. Wine, it is true, is not to be found in every village, especially where the inhabitants are not Christians. Now it often happens that the Christians, weary of Turkish insolence and contempt, withdraw from the main roads into more inaccessible parts, which are less fertile but safer, and leave the better land to their masters. Whenever, therefore, the Turks saw that we were approaching a wineless district, they would warn us that no wine would be obtainable ; and then our steward was sent a day ahead, accompanied by a Turk, to seek a supply from the nearest Christian villages. Thus my people were never without this alleviation of their hardships ; and wine took the place of soft mattresses and cushions and all the other appliances for wooing sleep. For myself, I had in my carriage bottles of a better brand of wine, and was thus well supplied. So there was always a provision of wine for myself and my followers.

There remained one annoyance, which was almost worse than a lack of wine, namely, that our sleep used to be interrupted in a most distressing manner. We often had to arise early, sometimes even before it was light, in order to arrive in good time at more convenient halting-places. The result was that our Turkish guides were sometimes deceived by the brightness of the moon and waked us with a loud clamour soon after midnight ; for the Turks have no hours to mark the time, just as they have no milestones to mark distances. They have, it is true, a class of men called *talismans*, attached to the service of their mosques, who make use of water-clocks. When they judge from these that dawn is at hand, they raise a shout from a high tower erected for the purpose, in order to exhort and invite men to say their prayers. They repeat the performance half-way between sunrise and midday, again at midday, and half-way between midday and sunset, and finally at sunset, uttering, in a tremulous voice, shrill but not unpleasing cries, which are audible at a greater distance than one would imagine possible. Thus the Turkish day is divided into four periods, which are longer or shorter, according to the time of year ; but at night there is nothing to mark the time. Our guides, as I have said, misled by the brightness of the moon, would give the signal for packing-up long before sunrise. We would then hastily get up, so that we might not be late or be blamed for any untoward incident that might occur ; our baggage would be collected, my bed and the tents hurled into the carriage, our horses harnessed, and we ourselves girt up and ready awaiting the signal for departure. Meanwhile the Turks, having realized their mistake, had returned to their beds and their slumbers. . . . I dealt with this annoyance by forbidding the Turks to disturb me in future, and undertaking to wake the party at the proper time, if they would warn me overnight of the hour at which we must start. I explained to them that I had clocks which never failed me, and would arrange matters, taking the responsibility of letting them sleep on ; they could, I said, safely trust me to get up. They assented, but were still not quite at their ease ; they arrived in the early morning, and, waking my valet, begged him to go and ask me 'what the fingers of my timepiece said'. He did this, and then indicated as best he could whether a long or a short time remained before the sun would rise. When they had tested us once or twice and found that they were not deceived, they relied on us henceforward and expressed their admiration of the trustworthiness of our clocks. Thus we could enjoy our sleep undisturbed by their clamour.

From Nish we journeyed to Sofia, both the weather and the road being tolerably good for the time of year. Sofia is a fairly large town with a considerable population of natives and foreigners. It was once the capital of the Despots of Bulgaria, and afterwards, if I remember right, of the Despots of Serbia, as long as their dynasty lasted and until it succumbed to the Turkish arms. After leaving Sofia we journeyed for several days through the pleasant, fertile valleys of the Bulgarians.

During this period of our journey we ate bread baked under ashes ; the natives call it *fugacia*. It is sold by girls and women, for there are no bakers in those parts. When they hear of the arrival of strangers from whom they hope to earn something, they hurriedly knead flour, mixed with water but without yeast, and put it under the hot cinders, and then bring the loaves for sale at a low price, still hot from the fire. All kinds of food are quite cheap ; a sheep costs 35 *aspres* (50 *aspres* make a crown), a cockerel or a pullet one *aspre*.

I must also describe the women's dress. They usually wear a single garment, a linen shirt or shift, quite as coarsely woven as our sack-cloth, and ornamented with clumsy and ridiculous embroidery, of which, however, they are inordinately proud. When they saw our shirts, which were of a very fine texture, they expressed their astonishment at our sober taste in wearing garments so plain and so devoid of colour and decoration. The most unusual features of their attire are their towering head-dresses and bonnets (if they can be so called), which are of a quite extraordinary shape. They are made of straw interwoven with threads, and in form are the exact contrary of those of our own peasant women, whose hats reach down to their shoulders and are broadest at the bottom and rise into a pyramid above. In Bulgaria they are narrowest at the bottom and then rise in a curve over the head to the height of about nine inches. Where they face the sky, they are very wide and open, so that they seem as well adapted to catch the rain and sun as our hats are to keep them off. From top to bottom they are covered with little coins and figures and pieces of glass of different colours ; and anything else which glitters, however worthless, is hung on as an ornament. A bonnet of this kind greatly adds to the wearer's height and also to the stateliness of her carriage, since it is easily dislodged by the slightest jar. So the women carry themselves as you would imagine that Clytemnestra would take the stage, or Hecuba while Troy still flourished.

I was reminded here of the fickleness and uncertainty of what men usually call nobility of birth. Noticing some girls who had an appearance of unusually good breeding, I asked whether they were the daughters of some great family. I was told that they traced their descent from the greatest rulers of the land and even from the royal house itself, but were

now married to ploughmen and shepherds. Such is
the lowly estate of nobility in the realm of Turkey.
Subsequently I saw elsewhere the descendants of the
imperial families of the Cantacuzeni and Palaeologi (*n*)
living in a humbler position than Dionysius at
Corinth (*n*) ; for in Turkey, even among the Turks
themselves, no value is attached to anything but personal merit. The house of Othman is the sole excep-
tion to this rule, being the only family in which birth
confers rank.

It is generally held that, when many nations were
migrating of their own accord or under compulsion,
the Bulgarians left the river Volga in Scythia and settled
here, and were called Bulgarians, that is Volgarians,
after that river. They settled among the Balkan mountains between Sofia and Philippopolis in a naturally
strong position which long enabled them to despise
the power of the Greek Emperors. They captured
in a skirmish and put to death Baldwin the Elder,
Count of Flanders (*n*), who had seized the throne of
the Eastern Empire. They could not, however, resist
the might of the Turks, who conquered them and
reduced them to a state of miserable servitude. They
speak the Illyrian tongue, like the Serbians and
Rascians.

Before descending into the plain in which Philippopolis lies, one has to traverse a pass over a very rough
mountain-ridge, called by the Turks ' Capi Derwent ',
that is, ' the Narrow Gate '. In the plain one soon
reaches the River Hebrus (Maritza), which rises not
far off in the Rhodopean mountains, the summit of
which, covered with deep snow, was visible before we
had traversed the pass. . . .

Philippopolis is situated on one of three hills, which lie apart from the rest of the mountains and look as if they had been torn away from them. While we were there we saw rice growing like wheat on wet, marshy ground. The whole plain is studded with tumuli, which, according to the Turkish account, are artificial, and were set up to commemorate the many battles which they say were fought in this region and mark the tombs of those who fell in the fray.

We followed pretty closely the bank of the Maritza, which flowed for some time on our right, leaving on the left the Balkan range, which extends towards the Black Sea ; then crossing the splendid bridge of Mustapha we reached Adrianople, or, as the Turks call it, Endrene. This city, before it received the name of Hadrian and was greatly enlarged, was called Oresta. It is situated at the junction of the Maritza, or Hebrus, and the smaller rivers Tundja and Arda, which from this point onwards bend their course towards the Aegean Sea. The extent of this city, as enclosed by the ancient walls, is not very great ; but it has spacious suburbs, the buildings of which, added by the Turks, greatly increase its size.

We stayed one day in Adrianople and then set out on the last stage of our journey to Constantinople, which was now close at hand. As we passed through this district we everywhere came across quantities of flowers—narcissi, hyacinths, and *tulipans*, as the Turks call them. We were surprised to find them flowering in mid-winter, scarcely a favourable season. There is an abundance of narcissi and hyacinths in Greece (*n*), and they possess so wonderful a scent that a large quantity of them causes a headache in those who are unaccustomed to such an odour. The tulip has little or no scent, but it is admired for its beauty and the variety of its colours. The Turks are very fond of flowers, and, though they are otherwise anything but extravagant, they do not hesitate to pay several *aspres* for a fine blossom. These flowers, although they were gifts, cost me a good deal ; for I had always to pay several *aspres* in return for them.

In fact, a man who intends to go among the Turks must be prepared, as soon as he has crossed the frontier, to open his purse and never close it till he leaves the country. Meanwhile he must sow money broadcast and pray that it may not prove unfruitful. If there is no other result, it is at any rate the only method of softening the fierce heart of the Turk, who hates all other nations. Money acts like a charm to sooth their otherwise intractable minds. Were it not for this expedient, their country would be as inaccessible to foreigners as those lands which are supposed to be condemned to perpetual solitude by excessive heat or cold.

About half-way between Adrianople and Constantinople is the little town of Tchorlu, famous as the scene of the battle between Selim (*n*) and his father Bajazet, whence Selim, thanks to his horse Carabuluk (' Black Cloud '), escaped in safety to his father-in-law, the King of the Crim-Tartars.

Just before we reached Silivri, a small sea-side town on our route, we saw clear traces of an ancient ditch and rampart which are said to have been constructed by the later Greek Emperors from the Sea of Marmora to the Danube, in order to include their territory within a line of defence and secure the estates of the inhabitants of Constantinople from the inroads of the barbarians. There is a story that an old man of those days declared that, in his opinion, the enclosure of this territory did not so much protect it against danger from the barbarians as mark the surrender of what lay beyond, with the result that it was likely to encourage an attack, while it discouraged the Greeks from defending it.

At Silivri the view of the calm sea tempted us to halt, and we enjoyed picking up shells and watching the shoals of dolphins, while the waves played upon the shore. The warmth of the air was delicious ; the softness and mildness of the climate defied description. At Tchorlu the wind was still rather chilly with something northerly in it, but afterwards the climate was wonderfully mild.

As we neared Constantinople we crossed by bridges over two lovely arms of the sea (*n*). It is a district the like of which for beauty could not, I think, be found anywhere, if only it were cultivated and art gave a little assistance to nature. As it is, the land seems to lament its fate and the neglect and scorn of its barbarian lords. Here we ate our fill of delicious sea-fish, caught before our very eyes.

While staying in the inns (which the Turks called Imaret), I often happened to notice pieces of paper thrust into the chinks of the walls. These aroused my curiosity, and I pulled them out, for I suspected that they were not placed there without some purpose. I took the opportunity of asking my Turkish friends what was written on them, but discovered that they contained nothing to account for their being thus preserved. This made me all the more anxious to dis-

cover why they were kept ; for I had often noticed
the same thing elsewhere. The Turks made no reply
and refused to tell me the reason, either because they
were ashamed to tell me a thing which I was unlikely
to believe, or else were unwilling to reveal such a
mystery to a stranger in religion. Afterwards, when
I grew more familiar with the Turks, I learnt from
my friends that the Turks have a great respect for
paper, because the name of God may be written upon
it ; so they never allow a scrap of paper to lie about,
and immediately pick up any that they find and thrust
it into some hole or cranny, in order that it may
not be trodden underfoot. With this practice you will
probably find no fault ; but listen to the rest of my
story. On the day of the Last Judgement, when
Mahomet summons the faithful to heaven from the
purgatory where they are being punished for their
sins, in order that they may partake of eternal bliss,
the only path which they can tread will be a huge
white-hot gridiron, over which they must pass with
bare feet. (You can imagine how painful this will be ;
picture to yourself a chicken hopping over hot embers.)
Then, wonderful to relate, all the paper which they
have preserved from being trampled underfoot in the
manner we have described will suddenly make its
appearance and adhere to the soles of their feet and
serve them well by preventing them from receiving
any hurt from the hot iron. So great is the merit to
be acquired for saving paper from ill treatment !
I remember on one occasion when our guides were
most indignant with my servants for putting paper to
an ignoble use, and reported the matter to me as
a serious crime. I told them that there was nothing

remarkable in such an act on the part of my servants, since they were also in the habit of eating pork !

So superstitious are the Turks that it is a terrible crime to sit down, even unwittingly, upon a copy of the Koran, their book of sacred law ; for a Christian it is even a capital offence. Also they never allow rose-leaves to lie upon the ground ; for they believe that the rose sprang from the sweat of Mahomet, just as the ancients thought that it came from the blood of Venus. But I must stop, lest I bore you with such trifles.

I reached Constantinople on 20 January. . . . The Sultan was away in Asia with his army, and no one was left in the capital except the Governor, the eunuch Ibrahim Pasha, and Roostem, who had then fallen from his high estate. Nevertheless, mindful of his former greatness and his hopes of a speedy restoration, we paid him an official visit and saluted him and made him presents.

It will, perhaps, not be out of place at this point to relate why Roostem was deposed from his high official position. Soleiman had had a son by a concu-bine, who, if I mistake not, came from the Crimea. His name was Mustapha, and he was then in the prime of life and enjoyed a high repute as a soldier. Solei-man, however, had several other children by Roxolana, to whom he was so much attached that he gave her the position of a legal wife and bestowed a dowry upon her, an act which is the surest pledge of a legal marriage among the Turks. In doing this he violated the custom of the Sultans who had preceded him, none of whom had contracted a marriage since the time of Bajazet I (n). Bajazet, having been defeated and having fallen, together with his wife, into the hands of

Tamerlane (*n*), underwent many intolerable sufferings, but there was nothing which he regarded as more humiliating than the insults and affronts to which his wife was subjected before his very eyes. Mindful of this, the Sultans who followed Bajazet on the throne abstained from marrying wives, so that, whatever fate befell them, they might not suffer a similar misfortune, and only begat children by women occupying the position of slaves, upon whom, as it was thought, disgrace would fall less heavily than upon legal wives. The Turks, indeed, do not think less highly of the children of concubines or mistresses than of those born from wives, and the former possess equal rights of inheritance.

Mustapha, on account of his remarkable natural gifts and the suitability of his age, was marked out by the affection of the soldiers and the wishes of the people as the certain successor of his father, who was already verging on old age. His stepmother, on the other hand, was doing her best to secure the throne for her own children, and was eager to counteract Mustapha's merits and his rights as the eldest son by asserting her authority as a wife. To effect her object, she employed the advice and help of Roostem, with whom her fortunes were closely linked by his marriage to her daughter, the Sultan's child ; so that their interests were identical.

Of all the Pashas Roostem enjoyed most influence and authority with the Sultan. A man of keen and far-seeing mind, he had been largely instrumental in promoting Soleiman's fame. If you wish to know his origin, he was a swineherd ; yet he was not unworthy of his high office but for the taint of mean avarice.

This was the only quality in him which aroused the Sultan's suspicion ; otherwise he enjoyed his affection and approval. Yet even this vice of his was employed in his master's interest, since he was entrusted with the privy purse and the management of his finances, which were a cause of considerable difficulty to Soleiman. In his administration he neglected no source of revenue, however small, even scraping together money by selling the vegetables and roses and violets which grew in the Sultan's gardens ; he also put up separately for sale the helmet, breastplate, and horse of every prisoner ; and he managed everything else on the same principle. The result was that he amassed large sums of money and filled Soleiman's treasury. . . .

The position of the sons of the Turkish Sultans is a most unhappy one ; for as soon as one of them succeeds his father, the rest are inevitably doomed to die. The Turks tolerate no rival to the throne ; indeed, the attitude of the soldiers of the bodyguard makes it impossible for them to do so. For if a brother of the reigning monarch chances to remain alive, they never stop demanding largesses ; and if their requests are refused, cries of ' Long live the brother ! ' ' God save the brother ! ' are heard, whereby they make it pretty clear that they intend to put him on the throne. Sultans of Turkey are thus compelled to stain their hands with their brothers' blood and to inaugurate their reign by murder. Whether Mustapha was afraid of this fate or Roxolana wished to save her own children by sacrificing him, it is certain that the action of the one or the other of them suggested to Soleiman the advisability of slaying his son.

The Sultan being at war with Sagthama, King of

Persia, Roostem had been sent against him as commander-in-chief. As he was approaching the Persian
frontier, he suddenly halted and sent a dispatch to
Soleiman saying that he was in a critical position, that
treachery was rife, and that the soldiers had been
bribed and were zealous for no one except Mustapha.
The Sultan, he added, alone possessed the necessary
authority ; he himself could not cope with the situation, which required the Sultan's presence and prestige ; if he wished to save his throne, he must come
at once. Alarmed at this news, Soleiman hurried to
the spot, and wrote summoning Mustapha, warning
him that he must clear himself of the crimes of which
he was suspected and now openly accused ; if he
could do so, no danger threatened him. Mustapha
was confronted by a difficult choice : if he entered
the presence of his angry and offended father, he ran
an undoubted risk ; if he refused, he clearly admitted
that he had contemplated an act of treason. He chose
the braver and more dangerous course. Leaving
Amasia, the seat of his government, he sought his
father's camp, which lay not far off. Either he relied
on his innocence, or else he was confident that no
harm could come to him in the presence of the army.
Be that as it may, he went to meet certain doom.

Soleiman before he left home had determined upon
his son's death, having first taken the advice of his
Mufti (who is the chief religious authority among the
Turks, as the Pope of Rome is among us), so that he
might not seem to have neglected the dictates of
religion. . . .

On the arrival of Mustapha in the camp there was
considerable excitement among the soldiers. He was

introduced into his father's tent, where everything
appeared peaceful ; there were no soldiers, no body-
servants or attendants, and nothing to inspire any
fear of treachery. However, several mutes (a class of
servant highly valued by the Turks), strong, sturdy
men, were there—his destined murderers. As soon
as he entered the inner tent, they made a determined
attack upon him and did their best to throw a noose
round him. Being a man of powerful build, he
defended himself stoutly and fought not only for his
life but for the throne ; for there was no doubt that,
if he could escape and throw himself among the
Janissaries, they would be so moved with indignation
and with pity for their favourite, that they would not
only protect him but also proclaim him as Sultan.
Soleiman, fearing this, and being only separated by
the linen tent-hangings from the scene upon which
this tragedy was taking place, when he found that
there was a delay in the execution of his plan, thrust
his head out of the part of the tent in which he was
and directed fierce and threatening glances upon the
mutes, and by menacing gestures sternly rebuked their
hesitation. Thereupon the mutes in their alarm, re-
doubling their efforts, hurled the unhappy Mustapha
to the ground and, throwing the bowstring round his
neck, strangled him. Then, laying his corpse on a rug,
they exposed it in front of the tent, so that the Janissaries might look upon the man whom they had wished
to make their Sultan.

When the news spread through the camp, pity and
grief were general throughout the army ; and no one
failed to come and gaze upon the sad sight. Most
prominent were the Janissaries, whose consternation

and rage were such that, had they had a leader, they would have stopped at nothing ; for they saw him whom they had hoped to have as their leader lying lifeless on the ground. The only course which remained was to endure with patience what they could not remedy. So, sad and silent, with their eyes full of tears, they betook themselves to their tents, where they could lament to their hearts' content the fate of their luckless favourite. First they inveighed against Soleiman as a crazy old lunatic ; then they railed against the treachery and cruelty of the young man's stepmother and the wickedness of Roostem, who together had extinguished the brightest star of the house of Othman. They passed that day in fasting, not even tasting water ; nay, there were some who remained without eating for several days.

Thus for some days there was general mourning throughout the camp ; and it seemed as if there was no likelihood of any end to the grief and lamentations of the soldiers, had not Soleiman stripped Roostem (probably at his own suggestion) of his dignities and sent him back to Constantinople without any official position. Achmet Pasha, a man of greater courage than judgement, who had occupied the second place when Roostem was Chief Vizier, was chosen to succeed him. This change soothed the grief and calmed the feelings of the soldiers, who, with the usual credulity of the vulgar, were easily led to believe that Soleiman had discovered the crimes of Roostem and the sorceries of his wife and had learnt wisdom, though it was too late, and had therefore deposed Roostem and would not spare even his wife on his return to Constantinople.

.   .   .   .   .

But I must return to my subject. A messenger was sent to Soleiman with a dispatch announcing my arrival. While we were awaiting his reply, I had an opportunity to see the sights of Constantinople at my leisure.

My first desire was to visit the church of St. Sophia, admission to which was only granted as a special favour ; for the Turks hold that the entrance of a Christian profanes their places of worship. It is indeed a magnificent mass of buildings and well worth a visit, with its huge vault or dome in the middle and lighted only by an open space at the top. Almost all the Turkish mosques are modelled upon St. Sophia. They say that formerly it was much larger and that its subsidiary buildings spread over a large area but have now been done away with, and that only the central shrine of the church remains.

As for the site of the city itself, it seems to have been created by nature for the capital of the world. It stands in Europe but looks out over Asia, and has Egypt and Africa on its right. Although these latter are not near, yet they are linked to the city owing to ease of communication by sea. On the left lie the Black Sea and the Sea of Azof, round which many nations dwell and into which many rivers flow on all sides, so that nothing useful to man is produced through the length and breadth of these countries which cannot be transported by sea to Constantinople with the utmost ease. On one side the city is washed by the Sea of Marmora ; on another side a harbour is formed by a river which Strabo calls, from its shape, the Golden Horn. On the third side it is joined to the mainland, and thus resembles a peninsula or promontory running out with the sea on one side, on the other the bay formed by the sea and the above-mentioned river. From the centre of Constantinople there is a charming view over the sea and the Asiatic Olympus, white with eternal snow.

The sea is everywhere full of fish, either making their way down, as is their habit, from the Sea of Azof and the Black Sea through the Bosporus and the Sea of Marmora to the Aegean and Mediterranean, or else on their journey up thence to the Black Sea. They travel in such large and densely packed shoals that they can sometimes even be captured by hand. Mackerel, tunny, mullet, bream, and sword-fish are caught in great abundance. The fishermen are usually Greeks rather than Turks. The latter, however, do not despise fish when they are placed before them, provided they are of the kind which they regard as clean ; they would sooner take deadly poison than eat the other kinds. I may mention in passing that a Turk would rather have his tongue cut out or his teeth drawn than taste any food which he looks upon as unclean—frogs, for example, and snails and tortoises. The Greeks entertain similar scruples. I had engaged a boy of the Greek religion to serve as a caterer in my household. The other servants had never been able to induce him to eat shell-fish, until one day they placed before him a plate of them so cooked and seasoned that, thinking that they were some other kind of fish, he ate most heartily of them. But when he learnt from their laughter and derision and from the shells which were afterwards shown to him that he had been deceived, you cannot imagine how upset he was. He retired to his chamber and indulged in endless vomiting and tears and misery. It would take fully two months' pay, he said, to atone for his sin ; for the Greek priests are in the habit of charging those who have confessed to them a greater or a less sum for absolution according to the nature and gravity of the offence, and will only grant absolution to those who pay them the price they ask.

At the end of the promontory, which I have mentioned, is the Palace of the Sultans, which, as far as I can judge (for I have not yet myself entered it), is not remarkable for the splendour of its architecture or decoration. Beneath the Palace, on lower ground, stretching right down to the sea, lie the Imperial Gardens. It is usually held that the ancient Byzantium lay in this quarter. You must not expect me to tell you why the people of Chalcedon, the site of which was opposite Byzantium and scarcely shows a trace at the present day, were called blind (*n*) ; nor about the perpetual and tideless current which flows down the Straits ; nor about the pickled delicacies which are brought to Constantinople from the Sea of Azof and are called by the Italians *moronella*, *botarga*, and *caviare*. All these details are unsuited to a letter, the limits of which I have already exceeded ; besides, they can be learnt from authors, both ancient and modern.

But to return to Constantinople. No place could be more beautiful or more conveniently situated. As I have already said, you will look in vain for elegant buildings in Turkish cities, nor are the streets fine, being so narrow as to preclude any pleasing appearance.

In many places there are remarkable remains of

ancient monuments, though one cannot help wondering why so few have survived, when one considers the number which were brought by Constantine from Rome. It is beside my present purpose to describe them in detail ; but I will mention a few of them. In the space occupied by the ancient Hippodrome two serpents of bronze (*n*) are to be seen, also a fine obelisk (*n*). Two remarkable columns are also to be seen in the city. One of them stands in the neighbourhood of the caravanserai where we lodged, the other in the market which the Turks call Avret-Bazar, that is, the Women's Market. This column is covered with reliefs (*n*) from top to bottom representing some expedition of Arcadius, who set it up and whose statue long surmounted it. It would be more accurate to describe it as a spiral than as a column, on account of the interior staircase which gives access to the summit. The column (*n*) which stands opposite the apartments usually occupied by the imperial representatives is composed, except for the base and capital, of eight solid blocks of porphyry so fitted together that they appear to form a monolith ; and indeed this is the popular belief. Where the blocks fit into one another there are laurel-wreaths surrounding the whole column, so that the joints are hidden from those who look up from below. This column, having been shaken by frequent earthquakes and burnt by a neighbouring fire, is splitting in many places, and is bound together by numerous iron rings to prevent it from falling to pieces. It is said to have been crowned by statues, first of Apollo, then of Constantine, and finally of Theodosius the elder, all of which were dislodged by gales or earthquakes.

The following story is told by the Greeks about the obelisk in the Hippodrome, which I have mentioned above. It was torn from its base and for many centuries lay upon the ground, until in the days of the later Emperors an architect was discovered who undertook to re-erect it on its base. When the price had been agreed upon, he set up an elaborate apparatus consisting chiefly of wheels and ropes, whereby he raised the immense stone and lifted it into the air, so that it was only a finger's length from the top of the base on which it had to rest. The spectators imagined that he had wasted his time and trouble on such vast preparations and would have to make a fresh start with great labour and expense. However, he was not in the least discouraged, and, profiting by his knowledge of natural science, ordered an immense quantity of water to be fetched. With this he drenched his machine for many hours, with the result that ropes which held the obelisk in position gradually became soaked and naturally tightened and contracted, so that they lifted the obelisk higher and set it upon the base, amid the admiration and applause of the multitude.

At Constantinople I saw wild beasts of various kinds—lynxes, wild cats, panthers, leopards, and lions. One of these was so well broken in and tamed that it allowed the keeper before my eyes to pull out of its mouth a sheep, which had just been given to it to eat, and remained quite calm, though its jaws had barely tasted blood. I also saw a quite young elephant which greatly amused me, because it could dance and play ball. I imagine that you will be unable to suppress a smile and will exclaim : ' What ! an elephant playing ball and dancing ! ' But why not, when Seneca

tells us of one which walked the tight rope, and Pliny
is our evidence for another which knew the Greek
alphabet ?   Now listen to my account, so that you
may not think I am inventing or misunderstand what
I say.   When the elephant was ordered to dance it
advanced on alternate feet, swaying to and fro with its
whole body, so that it obviously meant to dance a jig.
It played with a ball by cleverly catching it, when it
was thrown, with its trunk and hurling it back, as we
do with the hand.   If you are not satisfied from my
account that it danced and played ball, you must find
some one to give a clearer and more learned description.

There had been a camelopard (giraffe) among the
animals at Constantinople, but it had died just before my
arrival.   But I had its bones, which had been buried,
dug up for my inspection. This animal is much taller
in front than behind ; it is, therefore, ill adapted for
carrying a rider or a load.   It is called a camelopard
because it has a head and neck like a camel's and a
skin covered with spots like a leopard's.

If I had not visited the Black Sea when I had an
opportunity of sailing thither I should deserve to be
regarded as very lazy ; for to have seen the Black
Sea was regarded as not less difficult than to have
sailed to Corinth (n).   I had a delightful excursion,
and was allowed to enter several of the Sultan's
country-houses, places of pleasure and delight.   On
the folding doors of one of them I saw a vivid repre-
sentation in mosaic of the famous battle of Selim
against Ismael, King of Persia (n).   I also saw numerous
parks belonging to the Sultan situated in charming
valleys.   What homes for the Nymphs !   What abodes

of the Muses ! What places for studious retirement !
The very earth, as I have said, seemed to mourn and
to long for Christian care and culture. And even
more so Constantinople itself ; nay, the whole of
Greece (*n*). The land which discovered all the arts
and all liberal learning seems to demand back the
civilization which she has transmitted to us and to
implore our aid, in the name of our common faith,
against savage barbarism. But all in vain ; for the
lords of Christendom have their minds set on other
objects. The grievous bonds wherewith the Turks
oppress the Greeks are no worse than the vices which
hold us in thrall—luxury, gluttony, pride, ambition,
avarice, hatred, envy, and jealousy. By these our
hearts are so weighed down and stifled that they
cannot look up to heaven, or harbour any noble thought
or aspire to any great achievement. Our religion and
our sense of duty ought to have urged us to help our
afflicted brethren ; nay, even if fair glory and honour
fail to illumine our dull minds, yet at any rate self-
interest, the ruling principle of these days, ought to
stir us to rescue from the barbarians regions so fair
and so full of resources and advantages, and possess
them in their stead. As it is, we seek the Indies and
the Antipodes over vast fields of ocean, because there
the booty and spoil is richer and can be wrung from
the ignorant and guileless natives without the expenditure of a drop of blood. Religion is the pretext, gold
the real object.

It was far otherwise in the days of our forefathers.
So far from thinking that, like traders, they ought to
seek those lands where gold was most plentiful, they
went wherever the best chance was offered for show-

ing their valour and doing their duty. Honour, not self-interest, was the goal of their toils, their dangers, and their distant expeditions. They returned from their wars, every one of them, not wealthier in money but richer in renown. These opinions of mine are for your ear alone, lest haply any one should deem it a crime that I find anything lacking in the morals of the present age. However that may be, I see that the arrows are being whetted for our destruction, and I fear that in the future, if we refuse to fight for glory, we shall be obliged to fight for our very existence.

But to return to the Black Sea, or as the Turks call it, Karadenis, which means the same thing. It flows through narrow straits into the Thracian Bosporus, along which, buffeted against headlands, it reaches Constantinople with many eddyings and bendings in one day's journey. Then through an almost equally narrow passage it bursts its way into the Sea of Marmora. In the middle of the entrance into the Bosporus is a rock with a column upon it inscribed with the name of some Roman (Octavian, if I remember right). On the European shore is a high tower, called the Pharos, on which a light is burnt to guide sailors at night. Not very far away a little stream flows into the sea, in the bed of which we picked up pebbles hardly inferior to onyxes and sardonyxes ; at any rate, when they were polished, they were almost as brilliant. A few miles from the entrance is shown the narrow passage over which Darius led his army into Europe against the Scythians. About half-way down the Bosporus are two castles, one in Europe (Roumeli Hissar) and the other opposite on the Asiatic shore (Anatoli Hissar). The latter was held by the Turks before their attack on Constantinople ; the former with its strong towers was built by Mahomet some years before the storming of the city, and is used at the present day as a prison for distinguished captives (*n*). . . .

At this point you will perhaps expect me to give you some account of the floating Cyanean Islands, also called the ' Clashing Rocks ' (*n*). I must frankly confess that during the few hours that I spent there I could find no traces of any such islands ; perhaps they have floated away elsewhere ! . . .

One thing I ought to mention, namely, that Polybius was quite wrong when he argued on many grounds that in course of time the Black Sea would become choked by accumulations of sand owing to the alluvial deposits brought down by the Danube, Dneiper, and other rivers, and would thus be unnavigable. The Black Sea is not a whit less navigable than it was in his day. Thus time and experience often overthrow theories which no argument can refute. . . .

When the Sultan received the news of my arrival, a dispatch was brought to the Governor of Constantinople ordering that we should be conducted across into Asia and then sent on to Amasia. Accordingly, having made our preparations and procured guides, we crossed over into Anatolia, as the Turks now call Asia, on 9 March. That day we only got as far as Scutari, a village on the Asiatic coast opposite to the ancient Byzantium, at, or a little below, the site on which the famous city of Chalcedon is thought to have stood. The Turks considered that they had done quite enough travelling for one day in having conveyed us and our horses, carriages, and attendants across the straits. In particular they urged that, since Constantinople was still quite near, we could easily send back thither, if, as often happens, anything requisite for our journey had been forgotten or left behind.

The next day we left Scutari and journeyed through fields of fragrant plants, especially lavender. We noticed immense numbers of tortoises in this region wandering fearlessly about. We would have gladly caught them, if we had not preferred to spare the feelings of the Turks who accompanied us ; for had they touched them or even seen them brought to our table, they would have considered themselves so much polluted that no washing could possibly have cleansed them. I have remarked before upon the scruples which forbid both the Greeks and the Turks from coming into contact with animals of this kind. The result is that, since no one would snare so harmless an animal, tortoises abounded everywhere. I kept one which had two heads for some days ; and it would have lived longer if my carelessness had not allowed it to die.

The first day we reached a village called Cartali. It will be well if I give you henceforward the names of our halting-places ; the journey to Constantinople has been undertaken by many, but, as far as I am aware, no one in our days has traversed the route to Amasia. From Cartali we reached Gebise, a town of Bithynia which is thought to have been the ancient Libyssa, famous as the burial-place of Hannibal (n). It commands a charming view over the sea and the Bay of Ismid, and is remarkable for cypresses of extraordinary height and girth.

Our fourth halting-place after leaving Constantinople was Nicomedia (Ismid), a famous city in antiquity, where we saw nothing noteworthy except some
walls and fragments of architraves and columns, the
sole remaining traces of its ancient glory. The citadel,
which stands on a hill, is better preserved. A short
time before our visit a long wall of white marble was
brought to light by digging, part, I imagine, of the
ancient palace of the Kings of Bithynia.

From Nicomedia we crossed the ridge of Mount
Olympus and reached the village of Kasockli, and thence
journeyed to Nicaea (Isnik), where we arrived rather
late after nightfall. Hearing in the distance a loud noise
as of men laughing and jeering, I asked what it was,
thinking that perhaps some sailors—for we were near
the shores of the Ascanian Lake (*n*)—were jeering at us,
because, contrary to the Turkish custom, we were
travelling at night. I was told that the noise was the
howling of animals which the Turks call jackals. They
are a small species of wolf, larger than foxes, but quite
as voracious and gluttonous as ordinary wolves. They
go about in packs and are harmless to human beings
and flocks, obtaining their food rather by theft and
cunning than by violent methods. Owing to these
characteristics, the Turks call swindlers and cheats
' jackals ', especially if they come from Asia. They
make their way at night into the tents, and even into
the houses, of the Turks, and devour any food that
they find. If they can find no food, they gnaw anything made of leather, such as shoes, gaiters, belts,
sword-sheaths, &c. They are very clever at thieving,
except that, ridiculously enough, they sometimes
betray themselves ; for if one of the pack having

remained outside begins to howl, they all immediately do likewise, forgetting where they are. The noise then awakes the inhabitants, who snatch up their arms and take vengeance on the thieves thus caught in the act.

We spent the following day at Nicaea (Isnik), sleeping, I think, in the actual building in which the Nicene Council was held (*n*). Isnik lies on the shore of the lake of that name. The city walls and gates are well preserved. The latter are four in number, and are all visible from the middle of the market-place. They all bear ancient Latin inscriptions stating that the city was restored by Antoninus—which Antoninus I cannot remember, but he was certainly an emperor. Remains of his baths also exist, which the Turks were using as a quarry for public buildings at Constantinople. While we were there, they had discovered a fine statue, almost intact, representing an armed soldier, but they quickly mutilated it by blows from their hammers. When we showed our annoyance, the workmen laughed at us and asked whether we wished, in accordance with our custom, to worship it and pray to it.

Leaving Nicaea we came first to Yenishehr, then to Achbyuck, and then to Bazarjik, whence we journeyed to Boz-Euyuk (or Cassumbasa), situated in a very narrow pass over Mount Olympus. Almost all the journey from Nicaea to this point lay along the slopes of that mountain.

At Boz-Euyuk we lodged in a Turkish inn. Near to it was a rather lofty rock, high up in which a large square cistern had been hewn with a channel leading down from the bottom to the public road. The ancient inhabitants used to fill up this cistern in the winter with snow, so that, when it melted, it might flow down the channel to the road and provide cold water for the refreshment of the traveller's thirst. Public works of this kind are regarded by the Turks as the noblest form of alms, being of universal benefit to all alike. Not far from this place Otmanlik is visible on the right—the abode, I imagine, of the famous Othman, who first brought glory to the family of that name.

From this pass we descended into a broad plain, where at a place called Chiausada (*n*) we spent our first night under canvas ; for this seemed the best method of supporting the heat. Here we saw a subterranean building, lighted only by a skylight. We saw also the famous goats from whose fleece or hair—I avoid the controversy about goat's wool—is made the well-known cloth, known as camlet or watered cloth (mohair). The hair of these goats is very fine and wonderfully glossy, and hangs right down to the ground. The goat-herds do not shear it, but comb it out, and it is hardly less beautiful than silk. The goats are frequently dipped in the streams. Their food, which is the thin, dry grass of the district, is supposed to contribute to the fineness of their wool ; for it is certain that, if they are removed to other pastures, their coats change with the change of food, and their species is scarcely recognizable. The thread spun from this wool by the women of the district is taken to Angora, a city of Galatia, and there woven and dyed in a manner which I shall describe hereafter. In this country is also frequently found (indeed their flocks consist of little else) the breed of sheep with fat, heavy tails, weighing three or four, and sometimes even eight or ten, pounds. In the older sheep they sometimes reach such a size that they have to be laid on a little platform on two wheels, so that the sheep may drag what they cannot carry. You will not, perhaps, believe this, but it is quite true. While it cannot be denied that such tails may serve a good purpose on account of the fat which they yield, yet the rest of the meat seemed to me tougher and less tasty than our mutton. The shepherds who look after these flocks spend day and night in the fields, and take their wives and children about with them in wagons which serve them for houses, though they sometimes put up small tents. They wander over wide stretches of country, seeking out the plains, or high ground, or valleys, according to the time of year and the available pasture.

I think I discovered in this district several kinds of birds which have never been seen and are quite unknown in Europe, including a species of duck, which might well be called a ' trumpeter-bird ', so exactly does it imitate the sound of the horns blown by the conductors of posting carriages. This bird, although it has no means of defence, is bold and turbulent. The Turks even believe that it frightens away evil spirits. It is certainly fond of liberty, for after being kept for three whole years in a farmyard, when it has the chance it prefers its freedom to a liberal diet, and flies away to its former haunts in the beds of the rivers.

[Busbecq passes through a series of villages, crossing the river Sakariyeh (Sangarius), and reaches Angora (Ancyra).]

At Angora we remained one day. In view of the

great heat we did not hurry, and the Turks were of opinion that we had no need to do so ; for the representative of the King of Persia was still on the road, and they wished us both to reach Amasia about the same time.

In none of the villages through which we passed did we see anything at all noteworthy, except that in the Turkish cemeteries we often came upon columns and ancient slabs of fine marble, on which were remains of Greek and Latin inscriptions, but so mutilated as to be illegible. It gave me great pleasure, on arriving at each halting-place, to inquire for ancient inscriptions and Greek and Roman coins, or, failing these, for rare plants.

It is the custom of the Turks to fetch huge stones from a distance and use them for covering the tombs of their relatives, which would otherwise be exposed, for they do not fill them in with earth. Their object is to provide the deceased with a convenient place where he can sit and raise himself erect to plead his cause, as they believe he has to do, with his evil genius as his accuser and critic of his life on earth, and his good angel as counsel for the defence. A further reason for putting a heavy stone over the grave is to protect the corpse from the attacks of dogs, wolves, and other animals, especially the hyena, which is very common in those parts. It digs down into the tombs and pulls out the bodies, which it carries off to its lair, round which can be seen a vast heap of the bones of men, pack-animals, &c. The hyena is rather less tall than a wolf, but quite as long in the body ; it has a similar skin, but more bristly and covered with large, black spots ; its head is attached directly to its spine without any connecting joints, so that it has to turn completely round in order to look back. It is said to have a continuous bone in place of teeth. The Turks, like the ancients, attribute to the hyena a great potency in love affairs, and, although there were two hyenas in Constantinople during my stay there, their owners were reluctant to sell them to me, saying that they were keeping them for the Sultana (*n*), as the Sultan's wife is called, who is commonly reputed to retain his affection by love-charms and magic arts. . . .

We found everywhere a great abundance of ancient coins, especially of the later Emperors, Constantine, Constans, Justinus, Valens, Valentinus, Numerianus, Probus, Tacitus, &c. In many places the Turks use them as weights, especially for drachms and half-drachms, and call them *giaur manguri*, or ' infidels' money '. There were also many coins of the neighbouring towns of Asia, Amisus, Sinope, Comana, Amastris, and also of Amasia, the goal of our journey. A coppersmith, from whom I inquired for coins, greatly aroused my wrath by telling me that, a few days before, he had had a whole jarful of them and had made some bronze vessels out of them, thinking that they were of no use or value. I was very much grieved at the loss of all these relics of antiquity ; but I avenged myself by telling the man that, if he had still had them, I would have paid him a hundred gold pieces. I thus sent him away quite as saddened at so much profit having been snatched from his very grasp as I was annoyed at his destruction of ancient remains. . . .

Angora (Ancyra), our nineteenth halt since leaving Constantinople, is a town of Galatia (*n*), the former abode of a Gallic tribe, the Tectosages. It is mentioned by Pliny and Strabo, but the modern city probably only covers a portion of the ancient site.

At Angora we saw a very fine inscription (*n*), a copy of the tablets upon which Augustus drew up a succinct account of his public acts. I had it copied out by my people as far as it was legible. It is graven on the marble walls of a building, which was probably the ancient residence of the governor, now ruined and roofless. One half of it is upon the right as one enters, the other on the left. The upper paragraphs are almost intact ; in the middle difficulties begin owing to gaps ; the lowest portion has been so mutilated by blows of clubs and axes as to be illegible. This is a serious loss to literature and much to be deplored by the learned, especially as it is generally agreed that the city was consecrated to Augustus as a common gift from the province of Asia.

Here we also saw how the watered camlet (mohair), which I have already mentioned, made from the hair of goats, is dyed and given by means of a press its watered appearance from the ' waves ' produced by pouring water upon it. The pieces which have received the marks of very broad ' waves ' in continuous lines are considered the best and choicest. If the ' waves ' are smaller and of varying lengths and run into one another, though the colour and material may be the same, this is counted as a defect, and the cloth is valued at a price less by several gold pieces. The wearing of this cloth is a mark of distinction among the older Turks of high rank. Soleiman himself does not like to be seen wearing any material but this, and prefers a green colour, which, though to our ideas unsuited to a man of advanced years, is commended by their religion and the practice of Mahomet, their prophet, who even in old age habitually wore it.

Black is considered by the Turks a mean and unfortunate colour, and for any one to appear in black is unlucky and ill omened ; so much so that on several occasions the Pashas expressed their astonishment, and even seriously complained, because we approached them clad in black. No one in Turkey ever appears publicly in black raiment, unless he is the victim of serious financial loss or some other heavy calamity. Purple is held to confer distinction, but is regarded in time of war as prophetic of death ; white, yellow, blue, violet, and mouse-colour, &c., are considered luckier. The Turks indeed attach great importance to auguries and omens. It is well known that a Pasha has before now been removed from office because his horse has stumbled, this being regarded as portending some great calamity, which by his deposition from office can be transferred from the State to the private individual.

From Angora we journeyed to the village of Balygazar, thence to Zarekuct and Zermec Zii (n), whence we reached the banks of the river Halys (Kizil-Irmak). As we traversed this district toward the village of Algeos we could see in the distance the mountains near Sinope, which owe their red colour to the red ochre, which derives its name (*sinopis*) from that town.

The Halys is the famous river, formerly the boundary between the kingdoms of the Medes and the Lydians, about which the ancient oracle foretold that if Croesus crossed it to make war upon the Persians ' he would overthrow a mighty empire '—his own, though he knew it not. On its banks was a small wood, which at first attracted an interest as containing a strange kind of bush ; we soon discovered, however, that it was the liquorice-tree, and we took our fill of the juice extracted from its root. A peasant happened to be standing by, from whom we inquired through our interpreter whether there was an abundance of fish in the river and how they were caught. He replied that there were fish in plenty but that they could not be caught. On our expressing our surprise he explained that, if any one tried to put his hand upon the fish, they rushed away and did not wait to be caught ! . . .

The Turks are so frugal and think so little of the pleasures of eating that if they have bread and salt and some garlic or an onion, and a kind of sour milk, which was known to Galen (n) as *oxygala*, which they call *yoghoort*, they ask for nothing more. They dilute this milk with very cold water and crumble bread into it and take it when they are very hot and thirsty. We often experienced great benefit from this drink in the extreme heat ; it is not only palatable and digestible, but also possesses an extraordinary power of quenching the thirst. At all the caravanserais, which, as I have explained, are Turkish inns, there was an abundance of sour milk on sale as well as other kinds of relish. For the Turks, when they are travelling, do not require hot food or meat. Their relishes are sour milk, cheese, prunes, pears, peaches, quinces, figs, raisins, and cornel-cherries, all of which are boiled in clean water and set out on large earthenware trays. Each man buys what takes his fancy, and eats the fruit as a relish with his bread, and when he has

finished swallows the remaining juice by way of drink.
Thus their food and drink costs them very little—so
little that I dare say that a man of our country spends
more on food in one day than a Turk in twelve. Even
their formal banquets generally consist only of cakes and
buns and sweets of other kinds, with numerous courses
of rice, to which are added mutton and chicken.
Capons, however, are quite unknown to the Turks,
and they have never even heard of pheasants, thrushes,
beccaficoes, and the like. If there is a little honey or
sugar in the water which they drink, they would not
envy Jupiter his nectar.

There is one drink, however, which for complete-
ness sake I must not omit. They take raisins and have
them ground up, and, when they are ground and
pounded, they throw them into a wooden vessel. They
then pour over them a fixed quantity of hot water and
mix it in and carefully cover over the vessel and allow
the mixture to ferment for two days. If the process
of fermentation is too slow, they add lees of wine. If
you taste it when it is beginning to ferment, it would
seem insipid and disagreeable owing to its excessive
sweetness ; but afterwards it takes on a somewhat
acid flavour, and if mixed with something sweet it
is very pleasing to the palate. Thus for three or four
days it makes a delicious drink, especially if cooled
by plenty of snow, which is always obtainable in
Constantinople. They call it ' Arab sorbet ', that is
to say, the Arabian drink. It does not keep good for
more than this period and soon become absolutely
sour and affects the head and feet to no less a degree
than wine, and so comes under the ban of the Turkish
religion. I must admit that I found this kind of

drink very pleasing. I also found grapes, which they preserve for use in the summer, often wonderfully refreshing. The method of preservation, which I heard from their own lips, is as follows. They take a bunch in which the grapes are large and thoroughly ripe, a condition which is easily brought about by the heat of the sun in that part of the world. This they place in a wooden or earthenware vessel after first putting a layer of ground-up mustard seed in the bottom ; on the top of this they place the grapes and press them tight with a packing of the same mustard-flour round them. When the grapes fill the vessel to the top, they pour in unfermented wine, as new as possible, and fill the vessel up and finally close it. They allow the grapes to remain till the season of the year induces thirst and demands a remedy against drought and heat ; they then unseal the vessel and offer the grapes for sale together with the juice, which the Turks like quite as much as the grapes themselves. Personally, I found the taste of the mustard unpleasing, and used to have the grapes carefully washed ; I found them most pleasing and enjoyable in the great heats. The Egyptians had the preposterous custom of worshipping as deities the produce of their gardens from which they had experienced benefit ; so you must not be astonished that I gratefully sing the praises of those edibles which I found beneficial. But it is time for me to return to my journey.

From the banks of the River Halys (called by the Turks, I think, the Aitoczu), we reached Goukurthoy and then Tchoroum and afterwards Tekke Thioi. Here is a famous establishment of Turkish monks (*n*), whom they call Dervishes, from whom we learnt much about a hero called Chederle, a man of great physical and mortal courage, whom they declare to be identical with our St. George and to whom they ascribe the same achievements as we ascribe to our saint, namely, that he rescued a maiden by the slaughter of a huge and terrible dragon. They add many other stories and invent them according to their own pleasure, saying that he used to wander to distant climes and at last reached a river whereof the water gave immortality to those who drank it. They could not say in what part of the world this river was ; it should probably be placed in No-man's-land. All they could affirm about it was that it was hidden beneath a pall of dense darkness and obscurity, and that no mortal had managed to find it since the time of Chederle, who himself, freed from the laws of death, wanders to and fro on a splendid horse, who likewise had put off mortality by drinking of the same water. They say that he takes pleasure in battle and comes to the assistance of the righteous cause in the fight and of those who have implored his help, whatever their religion. The tales are laughable enough, but the following is still more deserving of ridicule : they declare that he was one of the companions and friends of Alexander the Great ! The Turks have no idea of chronology and dates, and make a wonderful mixture and confusion of all the epochs of history ; if it occurs to them to do so, they will not scruple to declare that Job was master of the ceremonies to King Solomon, and Alexander the Great his commander-in-chief, and they are guilty of even greater absurdities.

In the mosque, as the Turks call their shrines, is a fountain of the purest water constructed of splendid marble, which they would have us believe sprang from the urine of Chederle's horse. They also tell many tales about the companions of Chederle, his groom, and his sister's son, whose tombs they point out in the neighbourhood, and they tried to persuade us that many benefits are daily conferred by heaven on those who invoke their aid. The same superstition leads them to declare that fragments of stones and the actual earth on which Chederle stood while he was waiting for the dragon, if taken mixed in a draught are a sovereign remedy against fever and pains in the head and eyes. The whole region is full of snakes and vipers, to such a degree that, in the great heats, it is unapproachable by man owing to the number of the beasts who are basking in the sun. I must not omit to mention that the Turks are much amused at the pictures of St. George, whom they declare was their own Chederle, in the Greek churches, in which he is represented with a boy sitting behind him on the horse's haunches, and mixing wine and serving it to him ; for St. George is usually thus painted by the Greeks.

I am now approaching the end of a long journey ; there was only one halting-place, at Baglison, before we reached Amasia, where we arrived on the thirtieth day after our departure from Constantinople, namely 7 April. As we approached some Turks met us to congratulate us on our arrival and honour us by their escort.

Amasia is the principal town of Cappadocia, and the governor of that province usually holds his court of justice and has a stationary camp there. . . . It lies on two hills facing one another on either bank of the river Iris, which divides the city into two parts, so that from their slopes there is a view of the river as from the rising tiers of seats in a theatre, and one side of the town is completely visible from the other side. The hills approach one another so closely that there is only one road which gives entrance to and exit from the city for carriages and beasts of burden.

On the night of our arrival a great fire occurred, which the Janissaries extinguished by their usual method of pulling down the neighbouring houses. The Turkish soldiers certainly have reason to wish that fires should occur ; for since they are employed to extinguish them—usually, as I have said, by the destruction of adjoining buildings—they plunder the goods not only of those whose houses are burning but also of the neighbouring houses. They often, therefore, themselves secretly set fire to houses in order to have an opportunity for theft. I recall an example of this practice when I was at Constantinople. Many fires had occurred, and, though it was almost certain that they were not accidental, the incendiaries were not detected and the blame was popularly laid upon Persian spies. It was eventually discovered, after a more careful investigation, that bands of sailors from the harbour had caused the fires, in order that, under the cover of them, they might have an opportunity for plundering.

On the loftiest hill overlooking Amasia there stands a very considerable fortress which is held by a permanent Turkish garrison, either against the tribes of Asia who, as I shall explain later, are not very patient of the Turkish rule, or against the Persians, whose raids sometimes extend thither in spite of the great

distance. On this hill there are extensive remains of
ancient monuments, perhaps actually those of the
Cappadocian kings. Neither the houses nor the streets
of Amasia have any remarkable beauty. The houses
are made of clay on almost the same principle as is
employed in Spain. They have flat roofs of the same
material without any gables. If the roof is damaged
at all by rain or wind, they use the fragment of some
ancient column as a roller and move it backwards and
forwards, and thus compress and flatten the surface
again. In the summer the inhabitants sleep in the
open air on these roofs. The rain in this region is
neither heavy nor frequent ; but if it does rain, the
clothing of passers-by is greatly soiled by the mud
which everywhere drips from the roofs. I saw a young
satrap in the neighbourhood of our quarters dining on
a housetop reclining on a couch quite in the ancient
style.

On reaching Amasia we were taken to pay our
respects to Achmet, the Chief Vizier, and the other
Pashas (for the Sultan himself was away), and we
opened negotiations with them in accordance with
the Emperor's injunctions. The Pashas, anxious not to
appear at this early stage prejudiced against our cause,
displayed no opposition but postponed the matter
until their master could express his wishes. On his
return we were introduced into his presence ; but
neither in his attitude nor in his manner did he appear
very well disposed to our address, or the arguments
which we used, or the instructions which we brought.

The Sultan was seated on a rather low sofa, not
more than a foot from the ground and spread with
many costly coverlets and cushions embroidered with

exquisite work. Near him were his bow and arrows. His expression, as I have said, is anything but smiling, and has a sternness which, though sad, is full of majesty. On our arrival we were introduced into his presence by his chamberlains, who held our arms— a practice which has always been observed since a Croatian sought an interview and murdered the Sultan Amurath (n) in revenge for the slaughter of his master, Marcus the Despot of Serbia. After going through the pretence of kissing his hand, we were led to the wall facing him backwards, so as not to turn our backs or any part of them towards him. He then listened to the recital of my message, but, as it did not correspond with his expectations (for the demands of my imperial master were full of dignity and independence, and, therefore, far from acceptable to one who thought that his slightest wishes ought to be obeyed), he assumed an expression of disdain, and merely answered ' Giusel, Giusel ', that is, ' Well, Well '. We were then dismissed to our lodging.

The Sultan's head-quarters were crowded by numerous attendants, including many high officials. All the cavalry of the guard were there, the Spahis, Ghourebas, Ouloufedjis, and a large number of Janissaries. In all that great assembly no single man owed his dignity to anything but his personal merits and bravery ; no one is distinguished from the rest by his birth, and honour is paid to each man according to the nature of the duty and offices which he discharges. Thus there is no struggle for precedence, every man having his place assigned to him in virtue of the function which he performs. The Sultan himself assigns to all their duties and offices, and in doing so pays no attention to wealth or the empty claims of rank, and takes no account of any influence or popularity which a candidate may possess ; he only considers merit and scrutinizes the character, natural ability, and disposition of each. Thus each man is rewarded according to his deserts, and offices are filled by men capable of performing them. In Turkey every man has it in his power to make what he will of the position into which he is born and of his fortune in life. Those who hold the highest posts under the Sultan are very often the sons of shepherds and herdsmen, and, so far from being ashamed of their birth, they make it a subject of boasting, and the less they owe to their forefathers and to the accident of birth, the greater is the pride which they feel. They do not consider that good qualities can be conferred by birth or handed down by inheritance, but regard them partly as the gift of heaven and partly as the product of good training and constant toil and zeal. Just as they consider that an aptitude for the arts, such as music or mathematics or geometry, is not transmitted to a son and heir, so they hold that character is not hereditary, and that a son does not necessarily resemble his father, but his qualities are divinely infused into his bodily frame. Thus, among the Turks, dignities, offices, and administrative posts are the rewards of ability and merit ; those who are dishonest, lazy, and slothful never attain to distinction, but remain in obscurity and contempt. This is why the Turks succeed in all that they attempt and are a dominating race and daily extend the bounds of their rule. Our method is very different ; there is no room for merit, but everything depends on birth ; considerations of which alone open the way to high official position. On this subject I shall perhaps say more in another place, and you must regard these remarks as intended for your ears only.

Now come with me and cast your eye over the immense crowd of turbaned heads, wrapped in countless folds of the whitest silk, and bright raiment of every kind and hue, and everywhere the brilliance of gold, silver, purple, silk, and satin. A detailed description would be a lengthy task, and no mere words could give an adequate idea of the novelty of the sight. A more beautiful spectacle was never presented to my gaze. Yet amid all this luxury there was a great simplicity and economy. The dress of all has the same form whatever the wearer's rank ; and no edgings or useless trimmings are sewn on, as is the custom with us, costing a large sum of money and worn out in three days. Their most beautiful garments of silk or satin, even if they are embroidered, as they usually are, cost only a ducat to make.

The Turks were quite as much astonished at our manner of dress as we at theirs. They wear long robes which reach almost to their ankles, and are not only more imposing but seem to add to the stature ; our dress, on the other hand, is so short and tight that it discloses the forms of the body, which would be better hidden, and is thus anything but becoming, and besides, for some reason or other, it takes away from a man's height and gives him a stunted appearance.

What struck me as particularly praiseworthy in that great multitude was the silence and good discipline. There were none of the cries and murmurs which usually proceed from a motley concourse, and there was no crowding. Each man kept his appointed place in the quietest manner possible. The officers, namely, generals, colonels, captains, and lieutenants—to all of whom the Turks themselves give the title of Aga— were seated ; the common soldiers stood up. The most remarkable body of men were several thousand Janissaries, who stood in a long line apart from the rest and so motionless that, as they were at some distance from me, I was for a while doubtful whether they were living men or statues, until, being advised to follow the usual custom of saluting them, I saw them all bow their heads in answer to my salutation. On our departure from that part of the field, we saw another very pleasing sight, namely, the Sultan's bodyguard returning home mounted on horses, which were not only very fine and tall but splendidly groomed and caparisoned.

We came away from our audience with small hopes of obtaining what we demanded. The Persian ambassador had arrived on the 10th of May and had brought with him many splendid presents—carpets of the finest texture, Babylonian tent-hangings embroidered on the inner side in various colours, harness and trappings of exquisite workmanship, scimitars from Damascus adorned with jewels, and shields of wonderful beauty. But all these presents were eclipsed by a copy of the Koran, the book which contains their ceremonies and laws, which the Turks believe to have been composed by Mahomet under divine inspiration. A gift of this kind is very highly esteemed among them.

Peace was granted on the spot to the Persian representative, in order that greater attention might be paid

to us, with whom it seemed likely that there would
be more trouble. No possible honour towards the
Persian was omitted, that we might have no doubt
about the genuineness of the peace which had been
made with him. In all matters, as I have already said,
the Turks are in the habit of going to extremes,
whether in paying honour to their friends or in showing
their contempt by humiliating their foes. Ali Pasha,
the second Vizier, gave a dinner to the Persians in
a garden, which, though it was at some distance and
separated from us by a river, was visible from our
quarters ; for, as I have said, the situation of the town
on sloping ground is such that there is scarcely a spot
which one cannot see and in which one cannot be
seen. Ali Pasha, a Dalmatian by birth, is a delight-
fully intelligent person, and (what is surprising in
a Turk) by no means lacking in humanity. The Pashas
reclined with the ambassador under an awning which
shaded the table. A hundred youths, all clad alike,
served the meal, bringing the dishes to the table in the
following manner. They first advanced, drawn up at
equal distances from one another, towards the table
where the guests were reclining, with their hands
empty, so as not to hinder their salutations, which consisted of placing their hands on their thighs and bowing
their heads to the earth. After they had performed
this salutation, the attendant who had taken up his
position nearest to the kitchen received the dishes and
handed them on to the man next him, who passed
them on to a third ; the latter then handed them on
to a fourth, and so on, until they reached the attendant
who stood nearest to the table, from whose hands the
chief butler received them and placed them on the

table. In this manner a hundred or more plates streamed, so to speak, on to the table without any confusion. When this was accomplished, the attendants again saluted the guests and returned in the same order as they had come, except that those who had been last when they came were the first to withdraw, and those who were nearest to the table now brought up the rear. The other courses were brought to the table in the same manner. Thus in matters of small moment the Turks like to observe due order, whereas we neglect to do so in matters of the gravest importance. The ambassador's suite was entertained by some Turks not far from their master's table.

Peace having been, as I have said, ratified with the Persians, we could obtain from the Turks no terms which had even the semblance of justice. All that could be arranged between us was a truce for six months, during which an answer might be sent to Vienna and a further reply brought back. I had come to assume the functions of an ambassador in ordinary, but, since nothing had been arranged about a peace, the Pashas were resolved that I should depart to my royal master with a letter from Soleiman and bring back a reply if the King were pleased to send it. I was, therefore, again introduced into the Sultan's presence. Two ample embroidered robes reaching to my ankles were thrown about me, which were as much as I could carry. My attendants were also presented with silken robes of various colours and, clad in these, accompanied me. I thus proceeded in a stately procession, as though I were going to play the part of Agamemnon or some similar hero in a tragedy, and bade farewell to the Sultan after receiving his dispatch wrapped up

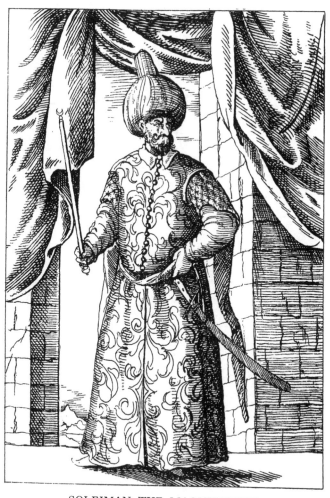

SOLEIMAN THE MAGNIFICENT

in cloth of gold and sealed. The more distinguished of my suite were also admitted to salute the Sultan. Having afterwards paid my respects to the Pashas in like manner, I left Amasia with my colleagues on June the 2nd. It is customary to offer a breakfast to ambassadors who are on the point of departing in the Divan, as they call the place where the Pashas administer justice ; but this is only done when they are friendly, and our relations had not yet been placed on a footing of peace.

You will probably wish me to describe the impression which Soleiman made upon me. He is beginning to feel the weight of years, but his dignity of demeanour and his general physical appearance are worthy of the ruler of so vast an empire. He has always been frugal and temperate, and was so even in his youth, when he might have erred without incurring blame in the eyes of the Turks. Even in his earlier years he did not indulge in wine or in those unnatural vices to which the Turks are often addicted. Even his bitterest critics can find nothing more serious to allege against him than his undue submission to his wife (n) and its result in his somewhat precipitate action in putting Mustapha to death, which is generally imputed to her employment of love-potions and incantations. It is generally agreed that, ever since he promoted her to the rank of his lawful wife, he has possessed no concubines, although there is no law to prevent his doing so. He is a strict guardian of his religion and its ceremonies, being not less desirous of upholding his faith than of extending his dominions. For his age— he has almost reached his sixtieth year—he enjoys quite good health, though his bad complexion may be due to some hidden malady ; and indeed it is generally believed that he has an incurable ulcer or gangrene on his leg. This defect of complexion he remedies by painting his face with a coating of red powder, when he wishes departing ambassadors to take with them a strong impression of his good health ; for he fancies that it contributes to inspire greater fear in foreign potentates if they think that he is well and strong. I noticed a clear indication of this practice on the present occasion ; for his appearance when he received me in the final audience was very different from that which he presented when he gave me an interview on my arrival.

We started on the return journey in the extreme heat of June, which was more than I could endure, with the result that I fell into a state of fever. It was accompanied by headache and catarrh, and, though mild and gentle, it was continuous, and only left me when I reached Constantinople.

The Persian ambassador left Amasia on the same day as ourselves, starting along the same route ; for, as I have already said, there is only one way in and out of the city, the ruggedness of the surrounding hills preventing any easy access on the other sides. This road soon divides into two, one of which leads to the east, and was taken by the Persians, the other to the west, which we followed. As we left Amasia we could see the Turkish camp with its closely packed tents extending in every direction over the wide plains.

I do not think that I need detain you by describing my return journey ; for we passed through practically the same places and halted at the same spots as in our way out, except that we returned more quickly, and sometimes went twice as far in the day. We thus reached Constantinople on 24 June. I leave you to imagine how trying the journey was to me suffering from continual fever. I arrived back in a much reduced condition ; but afterwards, thanks to the rest which I could take and the warm baths, in which I indulged on the advice of my physician Quacquelben, I easily recovered my lost strength. He also made me take a douche of cold water on leaving the bath ; though I did not enjoy it, it was most beneficial.

While I was at Constantinople, a man who had just returned from the Turkish camp told me a story which I shall be glad to record as illustrating how much the Asiatic peoples dislike the religion and rule of the Ottomans. He said that Soleiman, as he was returning, had enjoyed the hospitality of a certain Asiatic and had spent a night at his house. On the Sultan's departure, his host, considering his house to have been defiled and contaminated by the presence of such a guest, purified it with lustral water, much fumigation, and due ceremonial ritual. When this was reported to Soleiman, he ordered the man to be put to death and his house razed to the ground. Thus the man paid the penalty for his aversion of the Turk and his zeal for the Persians (n).

After remaining about a fortnight at Constantinople in order to regain my strength, I started on my journey to Vienna, the beginning of which may be said to have been ill omened. Just as we were leaving the city, we were met by wagon-loads of boys and girls who were being brought from Hungary to be sold in Constantinople. There is no commoner kind of merchandise than this in Turkey ; and, just as on the roads out of Antwerp one meets loads of various kinds of goods, so from time to time we were met by gangs of wretched Christian slaves of every kind who were being led to horrible servitude. Youths and men of advanced years were driven along in herds or else were tied together with chains, as horses with us are taken to market, and trailed along in a long line. At the sight I could scarcely restrain my tears in pity for the wretched plight of the Christian population.

If this is not enough to prove that I started my journey inauspiciously, here is another incident. My colleagues had entrusted to my care certain members of their retinue, who could not endure further residence in Turkey, that I might take them back with me. After two day's journey I noticed that their headman, who bore the official title of Voivode, was ill and rode in a carriage. His foot was bared in order to give relief to a plague-ulcer which was upon it. We were much troubled by this, for we were afraid that the contagion, as it usually does, might spread. He only held out against the disease until we reached Adrianople, which was not far off, and he there gave up the ghost. This led to further trouble ; for the rest of the Hungarians fell upon the dead man's belongings. One took his shoes, another his jerkin, another, for fear anything should be wasted, seized his shirt, another his linen ; and it was impossible to prevent them from exposing themselves, and us as well, to the most obvious peril. My physician rushed among them, begging them in heaven's name not to touch the clothing, since the infection would involve certain death ; but his words fell on deaf ears. As a result, on the second day after our departure from Adrianople these same men besieged my physician with prayers for a remedy against symptoms of headache and heaviness of the whole body accompanied by mental depression and dejection, which they suspected to be the beginning of the plague. He replied that his warnings had not been uttered without due cause, and that they had caught the disease, which they had done all they could to contract ; yet he would, he said, do his best for them, though he pointed out the difficulty of helping them in the midst of a journey, when no necessities could be procured. That very day, when, on our arrival at our quarters, we had gone out, according to our usual habit, to take a walk in search of objects of interest, I happened in a meadow upon a herb which was unfamiliar to me. I picked some leaves, and putting them to my nose and perceiving an odour of garlic, I handed them to my physician to see if he knew what the plant was. After a close examination he declared that it was scordium and, lifting his hands to heaven, he gave thanks to God for having sent so timely a remedy against the plague. He then collected a great quantity of the herb and threw it into a large vessel and put it on the fire to boil, at the same time bidding the Hungarians be of good cheer. He then divided the decoction amongst them, so that, when they were going to bed they might take it with Lemnian earth (n) and an electuary of dia-scordium, and he warned them not to go to sleep until they had perspired freely. They carried out his injunctions, and next day returned to him saying that they were better and asking for another dose. After drinking this they became convalescent. Thus by the grace of God we escaped from the terror of this foul disease. Yet even so we were not destined to finish our journey without mishap.

After passing through the countries of the Thracians and of the Bulgarians, whose territory extends to Nish, and of the Serbians, who stretch from Nish to Semandria, where the Rascians begin, we reached Belgrade in exceedingly hot weather, the Lion and the Dog-star being at their height. Here on the day appointed for fasting we were offered an abundance of excellent fish, including carp of great length and girth, which are caught in the Danube and are very highly esteemed. The members of my retinue gorged themselves with this fish, and owing either to their greed or else to the season of the year, many of them contracted fever. This huge quantity of fish, enough to satisfy forty persons, cost less than half a thaler, and almost every other commodity is equally cheap there. Hay, in particular, has no value at all ; any one can take as much as he likes from the fields, which are full of it, the only expense being the labour of cutting it and carting it away. After crossing the Save we could not but admire the good sense of the Hungarians of old who chose to settle in Pannonia, which is so rich in every kind of produce. We had traversed an immense extent of country both in Europe and beyond the sea, where the only grass, barley, oats, and wheat to be found was scorched and meagre and almost killed by drought ; but, as soon as we entered Hungary, the grass was so tall that it often hid the carriage in front from the one that followed—a clear proof of the excellence of the soil.

At Semandria, as I have said, the Rascians begin

and extend as far as the Drave. They are drunkards
and are generally reported to be treacherous. I have
been unable to discover their origin or the reason of
their name. They certainly showed much goodwill
towards us. After passing through several quite uninteresting settlements of theirs we reached the little
town of Essek, which is often cut off on almost every
side by marshes, and is famous as the scene of the defeat of Katzianer (n) and the destruction of our army.
Here, being unable to resist the heat by which we were
scorched as we traversed the wide, open plains of
Hungary, I was attacked by a tertian fever.

Leaving Essek we crossed the Drave and reached
Lasquen (n). While I rested there from the fatigue of the
journey and the exhaustion due to the heat and my
fever, the local officials came to congratulate me on
my safe arrival. They brought me enormous melons
and pears and plums of various kinds, besides bread
and wine, all of the most excellent quality—I doubt
whether even Campania, so renowned and celebrated
for the fertility of its soil, could produce anything
better. A long table in the room where I was resting
was loaded with these gifts. My retinue made the
Hungarians stay to dinner with them, making my
illness an excuse for not admitting them to my chamber.
When I awoke, my glance fell on the table, and uncertain whether I was awake or dreaming, I seemed to
see a veritable Horn of Plenty before my eyes. At
last I asked my physician whence these fruits had
come, and he told me that he had had them displayed
there that the sight of them at least might refresh me.
I asked him whether I might taste them ; and he did
not forbid me, provided I did not do more than taste

them. The fruits were therefore cut in slices and I tasted a little of each and was in no small degree refreshed. On the following day the Hungarians came and offered their services, and, after complaining of the wrongs committed by some of their neighbours, asked for the Emperor's protection.

From this place we came to Mohacz, the battlefield which saw the defeat of King Louis of Hungary (*n*). Not far from the town I saw the deep stream running between precipitous banks into which the unhappy youth plunged with his horse and so perished. I do not know whether it was by ill luck or ill judgement that he ventured to oppose the numerous and highly disciplined forces of Soleiman with a mere handful of hastily levied troops consisting mainly of unarmed peasants.

From Mohacz I came to Tolna, and from Tolna to Feldvar ; then I crossed on to a rather large island in the Danube, inhabited by Rascians, who call it Cophin. Then again crossing the Danube I reached Buda on August the 4th, the eleventh day after leaving Belgrade. We lost many horses on the way, who were choked by eating new barley and then drinking water which was too cold. We escaped many dangers from robbers, by whom the whole district is infested, especially Heydons. How narrow was our escape was subsequently shown by the evidence of some robbers who were punished by the Pasha of Buda. These men confessed that they had hidden in the bed of a broad stream which was spanned by a badly built bridge, in order to attack us from ambush. Nothing is easier than for a small body to surround a large party on a bridge of this kind. On account of the

rotten condition of the bridge and the gaping cracks
and holes in it you cannot cross, however careful you
are, without great danger of your horse falling ; and
if there are enemies to attack you in front and others
pressing on from behind, while your flanks are infested by others fighting in the bed of the stream and
hidden in bushes and sedge, while you yourself can
scarcely stir on your horse owing to the state of the
bridge, you are of course likely to come off worse
than the Romans in the Caudine Forks, and to be
captured or slain. I do not know whether our numbers
deterred the robbers, or the sight of the Hungarians
who accompanied me, or the fact that we were pro-
ceeding in a long column and did not all halt on the
bridge at the same time, or whether something else
frightened them ; but by heaven's grace we reached
Buda in safety.

[Busbecq has a somewhat unsatisfactory interview
with the Pasha of Buda, and journeys thence to Raab
and Gran. On the way a fracas occurred between his
Turkish advance guard and some Hungarians, who
seized a horse and cut off the nose of one of the
Turks.]

Thus we reached Gran, where, on the next day, the
Sanjak-bey gave me a kindly welcome and amongst
other things bade me remark the insolence of the Hungarian soldiers, who were not restrained even by the
presence of his royal majesty's ambassador from indulging their natural bent. He told me to make sure
that the horse which had been stolen was restored.
Meanwhile my Turk who had been wounded was
standing in the corner of the Sanjak-bey's courtyard
with his head all bandaged up on account of his nose,

which had been sewn on again, and emitting a hoarse and miserable noise and demanding that I should console him for his misfortune by a present. I said that I would give him enough to cure his wound, and presented him with two gold ducats. He asked for more, but the Sanjak-bey rebuked him, and declared that it was enough and more than enough to heal him ; he ought not, he said, to attribute to me a misfortune which was preordained to happen to him.

Then, after farewells, I journeyed that day to Komorn. I waited patiently for the recurrence of my fever at the usual interval, but discovered that it had at last left me and, being a Turkish fever, had not ventured to cross the frontier into Christendom. So I gave thanks to God, who had delivered me at the same time from the troubles of sickness and of a long and difficult journey.

Two days later I reached Vienna. I did not find my most gracious sovereign Ferdinand, King of the Romans, in residence ; in his place Maximilian, King of Bohemia, was there, and his kindness has caused me to a great extent to forget my past toils ; but even now J am so reduced by lack of comforts and emaciation and the hardships of my journey and illness, that many people imagine that I have been poisoned by the Turks. At any rate, when the Archduke Ferdinand was here recently and I went to pay my respects to him, he asked one of his attendants who I was, and the latter replied loud enough for me to hear that I was the man who had just returned from the country whence men generally returned in such a condition. He probably wished to suggest that, like Claudius of old, I had swallowed some sort of mushroom (*n*). But

I am quite sure that this is not so, and I have no doubt that, when I have rested awhile, I shall recover my complexion and strength and my general physical condition ; in fact, I feel a little better each day.

Meanwhile I have reported my arrival to the King of the Romans, and informed him of the six months' truce and given him a summary of my doings. When he returns home from the Diet, where he is now detained, he shall receive a detailed and more exact account of everything.

Many persons who were deterred by fear or some other motive from going with me to Constantinople would give a great deal to have returned with me. The line of Plautus (*n*) applies well to them :

He who would eat the nut must crack the shell.

A man is not justified in demanding a share of the profit, who has not taken his share of the toil.

I have now given you an account of my journey to Amasia as well as my journey to Constantinople—a coarsely spun yarn perhaps, just as I should tell it if we were talking together. It must be sufficient excuse for the style that I have written hurriedly in obedience to your request ; it would be hardly fair to expect from one who is in a hurry and very busy an elegance of diction which I could not guarantee even if I had time for careful composition and abundance of leisure. I shall console myself for these artless babblings by the consciousness that they are at any rate free from any taint of untruth, which is the greatest merit to be looked for in narratives of this kind.   Farewell.

THE SECOND LETTER

I HAVE received your letter in which you say that you
have heard of my second departure for Thrace (n), and
express your astonishment at my allowing myself to be
induced to revisit regions so notorious for the barbarity
and savagery of their inhabitants. You desire to know
how my journey went off, what condition of affairs
I found on my arrival, what reception I was accorded,
and, further, how my health is, whether I am enjoying
life, and what hope there is of my speedy return.
These questions you ask in the name of our old friendship, and here is my reply.

In the first place, the report which you had heard
of my return to these shores was quite accurate and
should not cause you any surprise. I was held by
my promise, and it was not open to me to refuse
a duty which I had undertaken once and for all. My
most gracious master Ferdinand, King of the Romans,
had appointed me ambassador in ordinary to Soleiman
for a period of years. The acceptance of this post, it
is true, appeared to depend on peace having been concluded ; since, however, hopes of peace had not been
entirely given up, there was no reason why I should
shun hardship and danger pending a definite decision
in favour of either a settled peace or open and declared
war. So, although I was perfectly well aware of the
danger which I should incur, and should have much
preferred to hand over my office to some one else,
yet, since I could not find a substitute, I had to yield
to necessity, namely, to the wishes of the most con-

siderate of masters. As soon as he had returned to Vienna from the Imperial Diet and had heard from my lips the story of my negotiations with Soleiman, he ordered me to gird myself up and be ready to start off, in order to take back dispatches to the court from which I had just returned.

It was winter, and the rain and the winds made the weather far from cheerful, when I was ordered to journey back to Constantinople with anything but good tidings in the dispatches which I was taking. It was, you say, putting my head again into the lion's mouth ; to which I reply that what is right once is right twice ; and surely, the greater the toil and danger which attaches to an honourable task, the greater is the glory and credit which it wins.

It was in November that I left Vienna in order again to traverse the long journey to the inhospitable shores of the Black Sea. I will not abuse your patience and weary you by detailing again the small incidents of travel—I expect that I already bored you by the story of my former journey—especially as we returned by practically the same route as we had previously followed.

I reached Constantinople at the beginning of January, having suffered the loss of one of my companions, who was carried off by an attack of burning fever due to the hardships of the journey. I found my colleagues safe and sound ; but great changes had taken place in the condition of affairs in Turkey. Bajazet, Soleiman's younger son, had freed himself from serious danger and was reconciled to his father ; Achmet Pasha, the Grand Vizier, had been strangled, and Roostem had recovered his old position of honour.

But of this more anon : I will first describe the unfavourable reception which I met with from the Sultan
and the Pashas and the Turks in general.

The Pashas, in accordance with their usual custom,
before introducing me into the Sultan's presence,
inquired of me what message I brought. When they
realized that the Emperor would not give up his rights
and claimed that the agreements should be observed
which he had made without force or fraud with the
widow and son of John, the Voivode or Governor of
Transylvania, they were fiercely and unreasonably
angry. A long period of success has made this people
so proud, that they regard whatever they wish as fair,
and whatever they do not wish as unfair. They,
therefore, began to threaten me and to dwell on the
great risk we should run if we entered the Sultan's
presence with such a message. When we, nevertheless, insisted on their introducing us, they said that
they would not involve themselves in our danger by
doing so. How many heads, they asked, did we
imagine that they possessed, that they should venture
to usher us into the Sultan's presence with such an
answer ? We were, they declared, obviously laughing
at him, and he would not bear such conduct with
equanimity. He was there with a victorious army,
and was inspirited and exalted by his successes against
the Persians ; the son who had set himself up as his
rival had been put to death—an act which showed
how far his anger would go. What better could he
wish for than to march his war-worn troops into
Hungary and recruit their strength on the spoils and
abundance of the inhabitants and annex to his empire
the small portion of that province which was still

unconquered. If we were wise, they said, we should keep quiet and not arouse the sleeping lion nor hasten on the troubles which were sure to come upon us soon enough. My conversations with the other Turks bore out these remarks of the Pashas. The most lenient treatment which they prophesied for us was that two of us would be thrown into a filthy dungeon, while the third, namely myself, would be sent back to his master with his nose and ears cut off. In addition, the truculent expressions and unfriendly glances which we noticed from those who passed our lodgings filled us with sad and gloomy forebodings.

Henceforward they began to use us more harshly and keep us in closer confinement, allowing no one to have access to us and never permitting us to go out, treating us in every way almost as prisoners instead of ambassadors. This has continued now for six months, and we have no idea what the future has in store for us. It will be as Heaven wills ; at any rate, whatever is our lot, we shall comfort ourselves in the thought that we are suffering in a worthy and honourable cause.

You wish for information about Bajazet, and here it is ; but, to make my account clearer, I must repeat what I have already said about Soleiman's family. He has had five sons, the eldest Mustapha, who was child of his concubine from the Crimea, and whose unhappy fate I have already described, and four sons by Roxolana, to whom he is legally married—Mahomet, Selim, Bajazet, and Jehangir. Mahomet married a wife (for the Turks bestow this title on concubines) and died young. Selim and Bajazet are still alive. The youngest son, Jehangir, died in the following circumstances.

When the news of Mustapha's death reached Constantinople, the unhappy youth, who was neither
mentally nor physically robust (he was disfigured by
a hump), was greatly alarmed, for he felt that a like
fate hung over himself. He could only hope to be
left unmolested as long as his father lived ; when he
was laid to rest, the accession of his successor, whoever
he was, would coincide with his own death ; none of
the brothers would be spared, but all alike would be
made away with as rivals to the throne, and among
them himself. These thoughts terrified him as much
as if his immediate execution had been ordered, so
that he fell ill and died.

Thus, as I have said, two sons survive ; one of
whom, Selim, being the elder, is destined by his
father to succeed him. Bajazet has the support of
his mother's zeal and affection ; either because she
pities him on account of the fate which inevitably
awaits him, or because of his dutiful attitude towards
her, or else because he has won her heart for some
other reason. Certainly no one doubts that, if the
choice lay with her, she would prefer Bajazet to Selim
and place him on the throne. But the father's wishes
must be respected, and he is steadfastly determined
that, at his death, no one but Selim shall succeed him.
Bajazet, knowing this, is seeking everywhere for some
means of escaping the doom which awaits him and
of winning a throne instead of certain death. The
support of his mother and of Roostem does not allow
him altogether to despair, and he deems it more
honourable to fall fighting for the throne and trying
his luck than to be butchered ingloriously, like a victim
for sacrifice, by the hand of his brother. Being of this

mind and already openly at enmity with Selim, he saw in the odium excited by the murder of Mustapha a not unfavourable opportunity of putting into execution a project which he had long entertained.

[Busbecq then describes how Bajazet induced his adherents to support the claims of a pretender who impersonated Mustapha and raised the standard of revolt in the Danubian provinces.]

Soleiman, rightly suspecting that the conspiracy was not taking place without the complicity of one of his two sons, decided that it must be taken seriously. He, therefore, wrote upbraiding the Sanjak-beys for having allowed the matter to go so far and for not having dealt with it at the very beginning, as they should have done. He threatened them with serious consequences if they did not send the impostor to him in chains at the earliest possible moment together with the other ringleaders of this wicked conspiracy. He added that, in order to facilitate matters, he was sending to their aid one of the Vizierial Pashas (namely, Pertau, who had married the widow of Mahomet (n), whom I have mentioned above), accompanied by a large force of soldiers of the guard ; if, however, they wished to clear themselves, they should finish off the business by themselves before the reinforcements arrived. . . .

The Sanjak-beys, on receiving Soleiman's orders, feeling that they must act with vigour, egged one another on and, setting to work with all speed, tried to checkmate and oppose the impostor's plans. They did their best to break up his bands as they were collecting and to scatter those which had already assembled, while they spread terror far and wide by threats of impending danger.

Meanwhile, the forces of Pertau Pasha were advancing. When they were not far from the scene of the rising, in accordance with the usual behaviour of half-trained troops who are suddenly surprised, the soldiers of the pretender, finding that they were being surrounded on all sides, were seized with panic. At first only a few slipped away ; but in the end, forgetful of their honour and their promises, they all deserted their leader and escaped as best they could. The pretender with his chief officers and advisers attempted to do likewise, but he was cut off by the Sanjak-beys and taken alive. All the prisoners were handed over to Pertau Pasha, who sent them with an escort of picked troops to Constantinople. There Soleiman had them strictly questioned under torture and learnt all he wished ; he discovered the guilt of Bajazet and all his plans. It was clear that it had been his intention, as soon as the insurgents had collected in sufficient numbers, himself to join them with a large body of men and, according as circumstances dictated, either to lead them straight against Constantinople or else to use them for a surprise attack upon his brother. Owing, however, to his hesitation, his plans were checked by the promptness of the Sultan before they came to maturity. Soleiman, having obtained all the information which he required, ordered the prisoners to be drowned in the sea at midnight ; for he judged that it was anything but expedient that any of the facts should be noised abroad or that his domestic troubles should be exposed to the eyes of neighbouring rulers.

Soleiman was greatly enraged against Bajazet, and was considering how he should punish him, and his wife, with her usual cleverness, easily read his thoughts.

Letting a few days elapse in order that his wrath might die down, she touched upon the subject in the Sultan's presence and dwelt upon the thoughtlessness of youth, and the inevitableness of fate (*n*), and quoted similar incidents from the past history of Turkey. She pointed out that it is a natural instinct in a man to do his best for himself and his family, and that all men alike wish to avoid death, and that a young man is very easily seduced by evil counsellors from the path of duty and rectitude. It was only fair, she said, to pardon a first offence ; and if his son amended his ways, his father would have gained much by sparing his son's life ; if, on the other hand, he returned to his evil ways, there would be ample opportunity to punish him for both his offences. She entreated him, if he would not have mercy on his son, to take pity on a mother's prayers on behalf of her own child. . . .

By these words, to which she added tears and caresses, Soleiman was softened, and, too much influenced, as always, by his wife, yielded and resolved to spare Bajazet, provided he came and received his orders in person. . . . When he entered his father's presence, Soleiman bade him sit at his side, and began sternly to upbraid his rash conduct in daring to take up arms under circumstances which made it seem probable that he himself was the object of his attack ; even if his schemes were aimed against his brother, his action must be regarded as an atrocious crime. He had, he said, done his best to root up the very foundations of their faith by endangering, through family feuds, the power of the house of Othman, which was the sole remaining support of the Moslem religion. . . .

He must cease henceforward from stirring up disorder and provoking his unoffending brother, and refrain from troubling his father's peace in his old age. If he returned to his old ways and raised a fresh storm it would burst on his own head, and there would be no pardon for a second offence ; he would find him not a kind father but the sternest of judges.

To these words Bajazet made a short and appropriate reply, deprecating rather than excusing his fault and promising obedience in future to his father's authority. Soleiman then ordered the usual beverage (a mixture of sugar and water and various juices) to be brought and offered to his son. Bajazet, not daring to refuse to drink, though he would have preferred to do so, drank as much as appearances required, in great anxiety lest it should be the last draught he should ever swallow. His father, however, soon put an end to his fears by drinking from the same cup. Bajazet, more fortunate than Mustapha in his interview with his father, then returned to the seat of his government.

[Busbecq next relates how Achmet was put to death and Roostem restored to the office of Chief Vizier.]

As to your inquiry about my return, you know the saying *Facilis descensus Averni* (*n*). But He who was my guide on my journey hither will guide me home again in His own good time. Meanwhile, I shall console myself for my loneliness and all my other troubles by communion with those old friends my books, who hitherto have never failed me, but always render me loyal and attentive service day and night. Farewell.

THE THIRD LETTER

THE news you have received is certainly correct
you know all the particulars ; my colleagues have left
me a long time ago and I have remained here alone.
You ask me what fatality or dire resolve kept me from
returning with them and bidding farewell to this
barbarous land and again enjoying the sight of the
native land for which I long. . . .

When my colleagues, with whom you are acquainted
from my former letters, saw that we had already spent
three years here in vain and that no arrangements had
been made for peace or a truce of any duration, and
there seemed only a vague and distant hope of making
any progress in the future, they began to exert all
their efforts to obtain leave to depart. When Soleiman
had with great difficulty been induced to consent to
their departure—for when a man has arrived here it is
no easy matter for him to return when he wishes to do
so—one question still remained, whether the others
should leave without me, since they had been here
longer than I, or whether we should all depart ; for
Soleiman, desirous of not appearing too eager for peace
by detaining any of us himself, left the choice to us.
My colleagues were of opinion that it was greatly to
the Emperor's interest that one of us should remain.
This was obvious (and I agreed with them), but
I thought it well to dissemble and hide my intention
from the Turks. And so, whenever the question was
mentioned in their presence, I expressed a strong
aversion to remaining. I admitted that I had come
as an ambassador in ordinary, but pointed out that
such a position was only possible when peace had been

arranged ; as long as peace was uncertain, I did not
see how I could remain without disobeying, or at any
rate going outside, my master's instructions, which
would be best carried out if we all departed. I argued
thus in order that, if I remained at the request of the
Turks, I might be in a better position than if I offered
to do so and forced my presence upon them. I fully
realized that, if we all departed, it meant not merely
throwing open a window whereby war might enter,
but throwing wide the gates of the Temple of Janus (n) ;
whereas, if I stayed, the prospect of peace was unimpaired. Before dispatches could be exchanged
between the two capitals, a long time would elapse
during which much might happen to render our
position more favourable. Finally, anything was
better than needlessly to make a terrible war inevitable. I was, however, well aware how little I was
consulting my own interests, since I was only preparing
trouble for myself and should have to support alone
a vast weight of responsibility ; and many various and
unforeseen circumstances were to be anticipated,
especially if my action resulted in a declaration of war.
But those who undertake such onerous duties must
think lightly of them in comparison with the public
interest, and must only look to what is for the advantage of the State. Roostem, by showing himself very
eager that I should remain, gave me greater freedom
of action ; he naturally realized how much it would
promote the outbreak of hostilities if we all departed
and the peace negotiations already begun were broken
off. He was particularly opposed to war at this time
with a foreign power, because, being a man of fore-
sight, he anticipated that, if Soleiman made an expedi-

tion into Hungary, his sons were sure to seize the
opportunity for some fresh attempt. . . . He, therefore,
summoned us to his house and detailed to my colleagues
at great length the arguments which he wished them
to place before the Emperor with a view to the conclusion of peace. He exhorted me to remain behind
and not to abandon the task which I had undertaken,
but to persevere until I had brought it to a successful
conclusion. He expressed his conviction that the
Emperor, who had never shown himself averse to
peace, would approve of my remaining at my post.
I, on my part, raised objections and refused to comply as far as I could conveniently and safely do so.
My remarks spurred on Roostem to further efforts
and, to prevent my putting an end to all hopes of peace,
he insisted that his master was very eager to lead an
army into Hungary, and would have done so long ago
but for the fact that he himself with the support and
help of the women (meaning his wife and his mother-
in-law) held him back, to use his own expression, by
clinging to the hem of his raiment. He begged us not
to provoke the sleeping lion and irritate him against
us. I, thereupon, became less vehement in my refusal,
and said that I would no longer refuse to remain, were
it not that I feared that they would immediately lay
the blame on me if anything occurred against their
wishes, though it was not in my power to prevent
this, and would vent their wrath on me. Roostem
bade me have no fear, whatever happened, that I
should be held responsible ; if I would but remain,
he would protect me ' as though I was his own
brother '. I said that I would consider the matter, and
so we parted.

The next day we were summoned to the Divan, which is their Council of State, where practically the same scene occurred, except that Roostem, in view of the presence of the other Pashas, spoke somewhat less openly. I eventually consented to remain, after depositing with the Pashas a written document in which I recorded that I was remaining without any knowledge of my master's wishes and therefore reserved every question free and unprejudiced for his decision ; I took nothing upon myself and denied responsibility for any result which Heaven might be pleased to ordain. This document proved afterwards of great service to me in times of difficulty, when anything happened to give the Pashas an excuse for dealing hardly with me. Such were the reason and the manner of my remaining behind.

My colleagues departed towards the end of August 1557. In the following winter the Sultan moved his court to Adrianople, according to his usual custom. His object was to threaten Hungary with invasion, while at the same time he was attracted by the opportunities offered for hawking and for enjoying a climate more bracing than that of Constantinople, both of which he regarded as beneficial to his health. Near Adrianople a large area of flooded country is formed where the rivers converge, abounding in wild ducks, geese, herons, sea eagles, cranes, hawks, and other birds. To capture these, he makes use of the assistance of small eagles, so trained that they make for their prey in the clouds and drive it down and seize upon it as it flies low, or else dash it to the ground by one frenzied swoop. I am told that he possesses falcons so well schooled that they are bold enough to attack a crane at the point where its wing is attached to its body, in such a way that they are safe from the blow of its beak, and thus force it headlong down. Their daring is not always successful, however ; for if they make the slightest error they are promptly punished by being transfixed by the crane's beak as by a dart, and falling lifeless to the ground. Such are the reasons why the Sultan is in the habit of repairing almost every year to Adrianople when winter comes on, and not returning to Constantinople until the frogs begin to be a nuisance with their croaking.

I was soon summoned thither by a letter from Roostem, who sent some horsemen to accompany me, and sixteen Janissaries, either as a mark of distinction or else to keep a watch upon me. Having been ordered to hasten, we journeyed by long stages, but, when we had only just begun our third day's journey, the Janissaries started to complain. They had to march on foot, and the road, as was natural at that time of year, was muddy ; hence they grumbled at having to traverse almost a double stage each day. They declared that they had never had to do this even when they were campaigning with the Sultan, and they could not endure it. I was troubled at this, since I did not wish to be hard upon them. As I was consulting with my people how I could get over the difficulty and make them more willing to travel, one of them remarked that he had noticed that they took particular delight in a kind of pudding which my cook concocted out of wine and eggs mixed with plenty of sugar and spice. ' Possibly ', he said, ' if this were served up to them every day for breakfast, they would bear the fatigue with more equanimity and show themselves more

amenable.' Strange as the suggestion appeared, I resolved to make the experiment, which proved a complete success. Soothed by the charms of the pudding
and cheered with plenty of wine with which to wash
it down, they were ready to start of their own accord,
and offered to accompany me to Buda, if they were
always so well treated.

Thus we reached Adrianople, where I had to listen
to the complaints, not to say abuse, of Roostem on
the subject of the raids and robberies of the Hungarians. I found a ready means of reply by pointing
out the frequent wrongs and numerous crimes from
which our people daily suffered at the hands of the
Turks ; what was there to wonder at, I asked, if our
people requited like with like ? A courier had arrived
most opportunely with a dispatch from the Emperor,
in which he drew attention to the way in which on our
frontier the Turks were daily violating the terms of the
truce, which we had concluded for a fixed period on
the departure of my colleagues, by harrying the unhappy peasantry by continual raids, laying waste their
property, and carrying off them and their wives and
children into captivity.

I must not omit to mention a serious earthquake
which occurred on the day on which this courier
reached Adrianople, in connexion with which he
related that he had felt a subterranean disturbance,
which he judged to be the same, at Nish and Sofia and
a series of other places through which he had passed ;
so that apparently the air enclosed within the caverns
of the earth had run a race with him and had traversed,
in almost the same period of time, the same distance
which he had covered on horseback. This theory was

confirmed by the fact that a similar earthquake occurred four days later at Constantinople, so that the same disturbance seemed to have travelled thither also. You can put what construction you like on these facts.

Constantinople is generally very liable to earthquakes. I remember an occasion on which, just after midnight, our lodgings began to shake with such violent motion that it seemed likely that they would fall in ruin. Awakened from a deep sleep I could see, by the night-light which was burning, a cup falling one way, a book another, a beam falling here and stones there, and the whole place shaking and tottering. For a moment I was amazed and dumbfounded by the strange phenomenon, until I realized that an earthquake was in progress, whereupon I took refuge where I hoped I should be safer from destruction. This earthquake lasted for several days, though not with the same violence. Throughout the city, but especially in the vicinity of our lodgings and St. Sophia, even in the most solid walls it was possible to see huge cracks caused by the disturbance.

I remained about three months at Adrianople, and was then conducted back to Constantinople in March after the conclusion of a seven months' truce. As I was tired of being confined in the same lodgings, I negotiated with my cavasse—a member of a class of officials, who, as I have remarked elsewhere, perform various duties amongst the Turks, including the custody of ambassadors—in order that I might be allowed to rent a house at my own expense, as the other ambassadors usually did, where I might have a bit of garden or a field in which I might breathe a freer air. He made no objection, seeing that a saving

would be effected by my paying myself for quarters
which hitherto the Sultan had provided at his own
expense at a yearly rent of 400 gold pieces (which
they call ducats), the amount of profit usually expected from letting a house. He was quite pleased
that his master should be relieved of this expense. So
I removed to a house, or rather block of buildings,
which I had hired out of my own pocket, with a considerable space of land about it, where I contemplated
making a garden and relieving the anxieties of my
official labours by cultivating it.

When, however, my custodian discovered by experience that in a house which was open and free of access
on all sides and surrounded by its own grounds it was
impossible to maintain so close a watch upon me as
in a caravanserai—a term, I think, familiar to you
from my former letters—which is furnished with barred
windows on all sides and has only one approach, he
changed his mind and arranged with the Pashas, who
had now returned from Adrianople, that I should be
again enclosed within the four walls of my former
quarters. However, I considered myself well treated,
since some of the Pashas held the view that, now that
I was alone, a less commodious and cheaper lodging
should be hired for me. The majority, however, were
more kindly disposed, and so I was taken back and
incarcerated in my old abode.

I should now like to make you better acquainted
with this dwelling of mine. It is situated on high
ground in the most densely populated quarter of
Constantinople. The back windows provide a delightful view over the sea in the distance, though near
enough to enable me to see the dolphins leaping and

sporting in the water, while far away the Asiatic Olympus can be discerned, white with perennial snow. It is open to all the breezes and is therefore regarded as a healthy place of residence ; the Turks, however, grudging such amenities to foreigners, not content with having blocked up the view by placing iron bars on the windows, have added parapets, which impede both the view and the free enjoyment of fresh air. This appears to have been done in deference to the complaints of the neighbours, who declared that they had no privacy from the gaze of the Christians. The building forms a perfect square with a large court in the centre, where there is a well. The upper story only is inhabited and is divided into a verandah, which runs all round, and dwelling-rooms, the verandah forming the inner portion and looking into the court. The rooms occupy the exterior part and all open into the verandah ; they are numerous but small, and all of the same size, like the cells in a monastery. The front of the building faces the street, which leads to the palace and along which the Sultan passes on his way to his devotions almost every Friday (which is a holiday like our Sunday), so that the ambassadors have frequent opportunities of seeing him from the windows. The whole household with the cavasse and Janissaries salute him from the entrance as he passes, or rather returns his salute, for it is customary among the Turks for the more important person to salute first. Thus the Sultan himself first bows to the people standing dutifully at the cross-roads, and they return his salutations with loyal applause and good wishes.

The ground-floor of the building is intended for stabling horses. The whole structure is rendered safe from fire by the interior arches upon which it is constructed and by a covering of lead which protects the exterior. In many respects the house is convenient, but it has several drawbacks. Everything is built for necessary use, and not for elegance or enjoyment ; there is nothing about it to attract one's attention by its beauty or novelty. It has no garden, in which one can take exercise, no tree or shrub, no greensward to rest the eye ; on the other hand, it is infested by various animals. There are swarms of weasels, numerous snakes, lizards, and scorpions. Sometimes, when you go in the morning to fetch your hat from the place where you left it the day before, you find it, to your great alarm, wreathed round by a snake. To give you my first instance of the wonderful ways in which we beguile our solitude, I must tell you that even these beasts provide us with a certain amount of amusement. Sometimes a weasel engages in a pitched battle with a snake and is not prevented by the presence of the whole household from dragging it victoriously to its hole in spite of its struggles and resistance. Sometimes a weasel changes its abode and transports its young ones elsewhere ; only recently, while I was still at my meal with some guests, one of these animals leapt down on to the middle of the table from its nest overhead, carrying one of its young in its mouth. When we had seized the latter, the mother left it there, but would not go far from the door, where she remained watching what would happen to it. Finally, when we had had enough of the ugly little creature, we put it down on the ground where she could see it ; whereupon she rushed up and caught hold of it and carried it off to her new abode.

Another curious phenomenon was a reptile, either a snake or a dragon, which had been trodden under foot by the horses in the stable ; its belly had a very swollen appearance, so I had it cut open and three large mice were discovered in it. I was puzzled how an animal which crawls so slowly could catch creatures who could run so fast, and swallow them down whole, although its jaws appeared so narrow ; I ceased to marvel when I came upon another snake which had seized in its mouth a very large toad, or poisonous frog, and had already swallowed a large part of it, beginning with its hind quarters. The toad was still alive and was struggling as best it could with its fore feet to escape from its enemy. At first sight I was greatly puzzled, thinking that it was some strange monster, namely, a two-footed animal with a tail as long as a snake. When I perceived what it was, I began to belabour it with a stick to make it give up its victim, but my efforts for some time produced no result. The snake tried to disgorge its prey, so as to escape more easily, but in spite of this the toad stuck in its throat, since it had sucked it in too far. When it was at last dislodged, the snake could not close its mouth, which remained open with a hideous grin in the same position until it was killed. The stick which I used, if Pliny is to be believed, would be useful to women in child-birth.

Not content with the creatures which are bred on the premises, I have filled the place with animals obtained elsewhere, the tending of which gives my household occupation and amusement, to my great satisfaction, and helps them to support with greater equanimity their longing to be back at home. For what better resource is there, when we are deprived of human intercourse, than to seek oblivion of our misfortunes in the society of animals ? What other amusement is to be had when one is isolated within the stone walls of a prison ? The monkeys are the first favourites, and cause much laughter with their wonderful tricks ; you can almost always see a group of bystanders watching with great amusement their wicked ways and ridiculous mischief. I also keep wolves, bears, flat-horned stags (often wrongly called fallow deer), common deer, young mules, lynxes, ichneumons, weasels of the kinds called martens and sables; also, if you care to know, a pig, whose society, according to the grooms, is very good for the horses. He must certainly be included in my list of animals, since many Asiatics visit my house on his account, in their desire to see this unclean animal, which their sacred writings forbid them to eat and which is banished from their land and, therefore, has never been seen by them ; indeed, all the Turks avoid contact with a pig as we avoid a man stricken by the plague. Realizing this prejudice, a friend of mine made good use of it, when he wished to send me a private packet, by making his servant take a little porker in the same parcel. As he entered, the cavasse asked him what he was taking in, and he whispered in his ear that he was bringing a little pig as a present to me from a friend. The cavasse poked the parcel with his stick, and on hearing a grunt, immediately retreated as far away as he could, saying, ' Get along in with you, you and your filthy present, bad luck to you ! ' Then spitting on the ground and turning to his co-religionaries, he exclaimed, ' It is extraordinary what delight these Christians take in this disgusting animal ; they positively refuse to be without it.' Thus the servant obtained admittance and brought me the packet which he wished to hide from the cavasse.

I also have numerous kinds of birds, eagles, crows, jackdaws, strange kinds of ducks, Balearic cranes and partridges. In fact my house is so full of animals that one of my friends has well compared it to Noah's ark.

My collection of animals, besides, as I have said, amusing my household and helping them to forget their long absence from home, also serves the purpose of enabling me to test the truth of many statements which I have read with incredulity in the writings of various authors, who give many instances of the extraordinary affection which animals have felt towards human beings. These I always refused to believe, for fear that I should seem too credulous, until I saw a lynx, which I obtained from Assyria, become in the course of a few days so attached to one of my men that it was impossible to deny that it had fallen in love with him. Whenever he was present, the beast would frequently single him out for caresses and embrace him and almost kiss him ; when he wished to go away, it would try to detain him by placing its claws gently on the hem of his raiment ; as he went away, it would follow him with its eyes, which it kept fixed in the direction in which he had departed, and would remain in a state of dejection until it saw him returning, whereupon it became extraordinarily lively and cheerful. It could not bear to be parted from him, and when the man accompanied me to the Turkish camp across the water, the lynx showed its grief by continual ill health, and after refusing to eat for many days, pined away and died. I was much annoyed at this, because I had intended to present

the animal, together with a very tame ichneumon, to
the Emperor, on account of the beauty of its coat, which
made it appear quite a different kind of animal from an
ordinary lynx. The most handsome lynxes come from
Assyria, and their skins are valued at fifteen or sixteen
gold crowns. . . .

Here is another story—this time about a bird.
Among the rest I have a Balearic crane, which differs
from the ordinary kind in the possession of a white
tuft of feathers drooping over each ear and black
feathers all over the back of its neck, with which the
Turks adorn their head-dress ; it also differs in size
from the common variety. This Balearic crane showed
the most obvious signs of affection for a Spanish
soldier, whom I had ransomed from captivity ; so
devoted was it to him that it would walk for hours at
his side, and stop when he stopped, and stand at his
side while he sat down, and allow itself to be patted
and stroked, while it disliked being touched by any
one else. When he was away from home, it would go
to his room and peck at the door with its beak by way
of knocking. If it was opened, it would look about
everywhere trying to discover him ; finding this to
be in vain, it would go all over the house with such
loud and piercing cries as to be quite intolerable, and
we were obliged to shut it up, so that its noise should
not offend our ears. When its friend returned, it
would spread its wings and rush to meet him with
such absurd and ungainly movements that it seemed
to be practising the figures of some outlandish dance
or preparing to skirmish with a pygmy (n). As though
this were not enough, it finally made a habit of sleeping
under his bed, where it actually laid an egg for him.

I have now given you two instances of affection shown towards man by animals ; you shall now have an example of the ferocity and treachery of an ungrateful creature. I had a tame stag, who lived with us for many months in a courteous and friendly spirit, but when the breeding season came round it suddenly became so savage that, forgetful of the ties of hospitality and past kindnesses, it declared war upon us and treated us as enemies, attacking every one with its horns and sparing none, so that we were obliged to restrain its rage by imprisonment and chains. One night, however, it broke loose and created a great panic among the horses, who, according to the usual Turkish practice, were left out at night in the open air of the courtyard. When the grooms rushed out to quell the disturbance and tried to make the runagate return to his prison, so far from allowing itself to be compelled, it wounded several of them. Excited by this they drove their foe into the stable, which, as I have said, is very spacious, and there, with my permission, pierced it through and through with spears and hunting-lances and any other weapon which was handy, and laid it low, though it put up a gallant and spirited defence in the face of vastly superior numbers, for it was beset by more than forty armed men. Thus it paid the penalty for its infraction of the laws of hospitality. I had it cut up and shared the results of the night's sport with all the ambassadors who were in Constantinople at the time. It was a stag of great size and bulk, resembling those which usually come up from Hungary into Austria at the beginning of autumn for the breeding season. I had obtained it from some beggars who made money out of it. They went about collecting alms, after first repeating a prayer in which the name of God frequently occurred, and on each occasion they bowed their heads and had trained the stag to do the same. The populace, delighted at its wonderful sagacity and imagining that it possessed a peculiar intuition of the divine, vied with one another in showering coppers upon its owners. I had intended, on account of its extraordinary size, to bring this stag back for the Emperor.

Now that I have mentioned Turkish beggars, it will not be out of place to give some account of them. They are far rarer than amongst us and are usually claimants to various kinds of sanctity, who wander from place to place, begging under the cloak of religion. Many of them pretend to be weak-minded as an excuse for their begging ; for persons of this kind always find favour with the Turks, who think that those who are half-witted and crazy, being certainly predestined to go to heaven, are to be regarded as saints during their life on earth. Another class consists of Arabs, who carry about standards, under which they declare that their ancestors fought in order to extend the Moslem religion. They do not beg everywhere or from everybody, but force upon passers-by in the evening a tallow candle or a lemon or a pomegranate, demanding twice or three times the proper price, apparently preferring to sell something rather than to incur the disgrace of begging.

But those who amongst us are beggars, with them are slaves, and if a slave becomes incapacitated his master still feeds him, and, however feeble he may be, it is always possible for him to make some return by working. I remember ransoming a Spanish soldier of some position, who had held a command in his own army ; though all his limbs were crippled by wounds, he had been purchased by a Turk, who discovered a means of making gain out of him, for he took him across into Asia, where large flocks of geese are reared, and hired him out to look after them, thereby making a by no means despicable profit.

I doubt whether the man who first abolished slavery was really a public benefactor. I am aware that slavery has various drawbacks, but these are outweighed by its advantages. If a just and mild form of slavery still existed, such as is prescribed by Roman law, particularly if the State were the owner of the slaves, there would not perhaps be need of so many gallows and gibbets to restrain those who possess nothing but their life and liberty, and whose want drives them to crime of every kind, while their freedom combined with poverty does not always lead them in the path of honesty. It is not every one that can endure want when he has full freedom of action, nor is every one endowed by nature with self-control and the ability to use his judgement aright ; hence the need of the guidance and direction of a superior, without which there will be no end to the crimes which will be committed, just as some animals will always be dangerous unless they are forcibly restrained by chains. In Turkey weak wills are controlled by the authority of a master, who, in return, lives on the labour of his slaves. The Turks both publicly and privately gain much from slavery and manage their houses economically by the employment of slaves ; hence the proverb which declares that no one can be regarded as poor if he possesses even a single slave. So, too, if the State requires any work of construction, removal, clearance, or demolition, slave-labour is always employed to carry it out. We can never achieve the magnificence of the works of antiquity ; and the reason is that we lack the necessary hands, that is, slave labour, to say nothing of the means of gaining knowledge of every kind which was supplied to the ancients by learned and educated slaves. However, please consider that these remarks are not meant very seriously.

Slaves constitute the main source of gain to the Turkish soldier. If he brings back with him from a campaign nothing but one or two slaves, he has done well and is amply rewarded for his toil ; for an ordinary slave is valued at forty or fifty crowns, while, if the slave has the additional recommendation of youth or beauty or skill in craftsmanship, he is worth twice as much. From this, I think, it is obvious what an enormous sum is made when five or six thousand prisoners are brought in from a campaign, and how profitable to the Turks such raids are. I note that the ancient Romans did not despise gains from this source ; their historians tell us that they carried off and sold by auction the entire population of towns, numbering 25,000 or 30,000 souls. An auction on this scale would bring in to the Turks about 150,000 crowns. However, they abstain from exercising the rights of war against men of their own religion, and never deprive them of their freedom.

But I must return from my digression. I have already told you about my hunting ; I must next say something about my fowling. While the Turks are indulgent towards all animals, they are especially so towards birds, and in particular towards kites, whose function, in their opinion, is to keep their cities clean. This kind of bird is, therefore, exceedingly common and, having no snares or weapons to fear, is almost tame. They come in answer to a whistle and seize in their talons fragments of food thrown into the air. It is my custom to order a sheep to be killed and to summon the kites to a public distribution of the intestines, pieces of which are hurled into the air. Immediately ten, twelve, twenty kites appear, and soon they are so numerous that they almost overshadow the house. Some of them are audacious enough to snatch the meat from the hands of those who hold it. Meanwhile, I stand behind a column with my crossbow and hit first one and then another on the tail or wings, as it may chance, with clay pellets, until I bring down one or two of them by a mortal blow. I only venture to do this with the gates bolted, so as not to annoy the Turks.

While I am on the subject of birds, I must not forget to tell you about my partridges, so that you may have a complete account of my amusements and perhaps be as surprised as I was at their behaviour. I had them brought from Chios, and they belonged to the species which has red beaks and legs. They were so tame as to be a positive nuisance ; they were continually hanging round my feet, pecking at my satin slippers in order to powder themselves with dust. They were so tiresome that I had them shut up in a room, where they all died in a few days of overfeeding, if I am to believe the story told by my attendants. Pliny, however, declares somewhere that hares and partridges never grow fat. So far there is nothing extraordinary ; but listen to the rest of my story.

Chios is full of these birds, who live in the houses
with their owners. Almost every peasant keeps a large
or small number of them, according to his inclination
or circumstances. At early dawn the public herdsman
summons them by whistling, and they all rush forth
and congregate in the street. They then follow the
herdsman, as sheep do with us, and proceed to a field,
where they pass the whole day basking in the sun and
feeding. In the evening, summoned by the same
signal, they form up and betake themselves home to
their familiar quarters. It is said that this habit is
formed because the peasants, as soon as the young are
hatched, place them in their bosoms inside their
shirts and carry them about and nurse them there for
a day or two, and put them from time to time to their
lips and feed them with saliva. Like most animals,
they have better memories and are more grateful than
human beings, and this kind treatment binds them to
their owners, whom they never forget. One precau-
tion, however, has to be observed, namely, that they
must never be left out at night ; for if this happens
once or twice, they promptly revert to a state of nature,
preferring a life of freedom to living in human com-
panionship. I am very anxious to bring back a skilful
partridge-tamer for the Emperor, that he may introduce amongst us this method of keeping partridges.
I have not actually seen the method at work, but I have
been informed about it by so many reliable witnesses
that I believe their accounts as though I had seen it
with my own eyes. The same is true also of the
following story, which is so widely reported and
generally admitted to be true that he would be thought
a fool who ventured to throw any doubt upon it. Those

who come hither from Egypt—and many come continually—constantly affirm that there eggs are not put
under hens, as they are with us, but certain men,
whose duty it is, construct in the spring a kind of
oven, made of heaped-up manure and dung, to which
the whole neighbourhood brings its eggs from far and
wide. In this oven the eggs are quickened by the
heat of the sun and of the rotting dung, and in due
time produce chickens, which are handed back to the
persons who brought the eggs by those who superin-
tend the business, who do not count them (for this
would be too long a task) but weigh them out. . . .

I have a number of thoroughbred horses, Syrian,
Cilician, Arabian, and Cappadocian, also baggage-
camels, and everything else ready for my return
journey ; for I want the Turks to believe that I have
carried out all my master's behests and am only waiting for permission to depart. This I have long been
urgently demanding, for, in view of the existing
quarrels and civil war between the royal princes, I do
not despair of obtaining tolerable conditions of peace.

I take great pleasure in watching my horses, speci-
ally in the summer months, when, in the evening,
they are all brought out of their stable and picketed
in the court, to enjoy the night breezes and rest more
at their ease. They come out and show their delight
by prancing and throwing up their heads and tossing
their manes, so that they seem conscious that they are
being watched. Their fore feet are hobbled, and one
of their hind legs is attached by a rope to a stake.
No horses are tamer than the Turkish or so readily
recognize their master and the groom who looks after
them ; so kind is the treatment bestowed on them

while they are being trained. On my journey to
Cappadocia through the region of Pontus and the part
of Bithynia which is called from its condition Axylus
(woodless), I noticed what care the peasants bestowed
on the colts while they were young and tender, how
they petted them and admitted them to their houses and
almost to their tables, and stroked and caressed them ;
you might say that they almost counted them among
their children. They all wear round their necks a kind
of collar, consisting of rows of amulets against the evil
eye, which is greatly dreaded. The grooms who are
in charge of them are equally kind to them, winning
their affection by constantly patting them and never
venting their rage upon them with a stick unless
absolutely compelled to do so. The result is that they
become most affectionate towards man, while you will
never come across a horse which kicks or bites or is
refractory, viciousness of this kind being exceedingly
rare. By heaven, how different are our methods ! Our
stable men think that no effect is produced unless they
are always bawling at their horses and continually
belabouring their flanks ; with the result that the
horses tremble all over with fear, whenever the grooms
enter the stable, and equally loathe and fear them.
The Turks like to train their horses to kneel down at
the word of command and allow their master to mount,
and to pick up a walking-stick, cudgel, or sword in
their teeth from the ground and give it to the rider
on their back. When they have learnt these accom-
plishments, they place silver rings in their nostrils as
a mark of distinction and a proof that they are pro-
perly trained. I have noticed horses who stood quite
still when their master had been thrown from the

saddle ; others who would circle round their groom, who stood at a distance, and halt at his command ; and others who, while their master was dining with me in an upper room, stood with their ears pricked listening for his voice and whinnying when they heard it. It is a peculiar characteristic of Turkish horses that they always come to a standstill with their necks stretched stiffly out and cannot stop or turn in a narrow space ; this is the fault, if I may so call it, of the bit, which everywhere in Turkey is of the same kind and shape, and is not made tighter or looser, as with us, to suit the horse's mouth. Turkish horses are shod with shoes which are not so open in the middle as ours, but are almost continuous and solid, so that their feet are less likely to be damaged by stumbling. They live considerably longer than with us, and one sees twenty-year-old horses as spirited and strong as our eight-year-olds : some, whose services have won them their keep for the rest of their lives in the Sultan's stables, are said to have lived to fifty years or even longer. On summer nights, when the heat is intense, they do not keep the horses under cover, but expose them, as I have said, to the night breezes, covering them with horse-rugs and giving them a litter of dry dung. For this purpose they collect the horses' droppings all through the year and dry them in the sun and break them up and reduce them to powder. They use it for the horses' bedding, and indeed know of no other kind. Of straw they make no use, not even for food ; but they give them a little hay and a moderate quantity of barley, which nourishes rather than fattens them ; for they like their animals to be rather thin, considering that they are thus fitter for long journeys and labour of every kind. The horse-cloths which I mentioned are put on in summer just as in winter, but they vary them according to the weather. They consider that to keep them covered both conduces to sleekness of coat and is a necessary protection against the cold, since they are sensitive to chill, and, in particular, suffer from exposure to bad weather.

As I have already remarked, I take pleasure in watching my horses towards sunset when they are picketed each in its proper place in the court, and when I call them by name—' Arab ' or ' Caraman ' or whatever they are called—they reply by whinnying and look towards me. For I make a practice of going down to them from time to time and distributing melon skins amongst them with my own hands ; hence the notice which they take of me. Indeed, I seek by whatever means I can to forget the annoyances which beset me.

I have six female camels, which I have bought to carry baggage ; but my real object is to take them back for my royal masters, in the hope that they may be induced by the consideration of their usefulness to breed this kind of animal. There are two things from which, in my opinion, the Turks derive the greatest advantage and profit, rice among cereals and camels among beasts of burden ; both are admirably adapted to the distant campaigns which they wage. Rice keeps well and provides a wholesome food, a little of which suffices to feed a large number. Camels can carry very heavy burdens, endure hunger and thirst, and require very little attention. One driver is enough to look after six camels ; and no animal is more amenable to discipline. The camel does not require combing or scraping, but, like one's clothes, can be kept clean by brushing. They lie, or, to be more accurate, kneel on the bare ground and allow themselves to be loaded. If the burden is heavier than they can reasonably carry, they protest by grunting and refuse to get up. They are apt, however, to rupture themselves if their load is too heavy, especially if the road be muddy or slippery. It is a pleasure to see how they kneel in a circle with their heads close together, eating and drinking with the utmost goodwill out of the same manger or basin, content with the scantiest fare. If necessary, owing to lack of fodder, they chew up brambles and thorns, and the more these make their mouths bleed the more they are pleased. Some of these camels are supplied from Scythia, but the majority come from Sinai and Assyria, where they are fed in great herds, and are so plentiful and cheap that a well-bred mare is sometimes exchanged for a hundred camels. It is not, however, the cheapness of the camel which perhaps should call for our wonder so much as the dearness of the mare and the price asked for it ; for mares of this kind are so highly esteemed that one who possesses even one of them regards himself as a man of wealth. The test of their excellence consists in their being ridden at a breakneck speed down a steep mountain-side without stumbling.

The Sultan, when he sets out on a campaign, takes as many as 40,000 camels with him, and almost as many baggage-mules, most of whom, if his destination is Persia, are loaded with cereals of every kind, especially rice. Mules and camels are also employed to carry tents and arms and warlike machines and implements of every kind. The territories called Persia which are ruled by the Sophi, as we call him (the

Turkish name being Kizilbash), are much less fertile than our country ; and, further, it is the custom of the inhabitants, when their land is invaded, to lay waste and burn everything, and so force the enemy to retire through lack of food. The latter, therefore, are faced with serious peril, unless they bring an abundance of food with them. They are careful, however, to avoid touching the supplies which they carry with them as long as they are marching against their foes, but reserve them, as far as possible, for their return journey, when the moment for retirement comes and they are forced to retrace their steps through regions which the enemy has laid waste, or which the immense multitude of men and baggage animals has, as it were, scraped bare, like a swarm of locusts. It is only then that the Sultan's store of provisions is opened, and just enough food to sustain life is weighed out each day to the Janissaries and the other troops in attendance upon him. The other soldiers are badly off, if they have not provided food for their own use ; most of them, having often experienced such difficulties during their campaigns—and this is particularly true of the cavalry—take a horse on a leading-rein loaded with many of the necessities of life. These include a small piece of canvas to use as a tent, which may protect them from the sun or a shower of rain, also some clothing and bedding and a private store of provisions, consisting of a leather sack or two of the finest flour, a small jar of butter, and some spices and salt ; on these they support life when they are reduced to the extremes of hunger. They take a few spoonfuls of flour and place them in water, adding a little butter, and then flavour the mixture with salt and spices. This, when it is put on the fire, boils and swells up so as to fill a large bowl. They eat of it once or twice a day, according to the quantity, without any bread, unless they have with them some toasted bread or biscuit. They thus contrive to live on short rations for a month or even longer, if necessary. Some soldiers take with them a little sack full of beef dried and reduced to a powder, which they employ in the same manner as the flour, and which is of great benefit as a more solid form of nourishment. Sometimes, too, they have recourse to horseflesh ; for in a great army a large number of horses necessarily dies, and any that die in good condition furnish a welcome meal to men who are starving. I may add that men whose horses have died, when the Sultan moves his camp, stand in a long row on the road by which he is to pass with their harness or saddles on their heads, as a sign that they have lost their horses, and implore his help to purchase others. The Sultan then assists them with whatever gift he thinks fit.

All this will show you with what patience, sobriety, and economy the Turks struggle against the difficulties which beset them, and wait for better times. How different are our soldiers, who on campaign despise ordinary food and expect dainty dishes (such as thrushes and beccaficoes) and elaborate meals. If these are not supplied, they mutiny and cause their own ruin ; and even if they are supplied, they ruin themselves just the same. For each man is his own worst enemy and has no more deadly foe than his own intemperance, which kills him if the enemy is slow to do so. I tremble when I think of what the future must bring when I compare the Turkish system with

our own ; one army must prevail and the other be
destroyed, for certainly both cannot remain unscathed.
On their side are the resources of a mighty empire,
strength unimpaired, experience and practice in fighting, a veteran soldiery, habituation to victory, endurance of toil, unity, order, discipline, frugality, and
watchfulness. On our side is public poverty, private
luxury, impaired strength, broken spirit, lack of
endurance and training ; the soldiers are insubor-
dinate, the officers avaricious ; there is contempt for
discipline ; licence, recklessness, drunkenness, and
debauchery are rife ; and, worst of all, the enemy is
accustomed to victory, and we to defeat. Can we doubt
what the result will be ? Persia alone interposes in
our favour ; for the enemy, as he hastens to attack,
must keep an eye on this menace in his rear. But
Persia is only delaying our fate ; it cannot save us.
When the Turks have settled with Persia, they will
fly at our throats supported by the might of the whole
East ; how unprepared we are I dare not say !

But to return to the point from which I digressed.
I mentioned that baggage animals are employed on
campaign to carry the arms and tents, which mainly
belong to the Janissaries. The Turks take the utmost
care to keep their soldiers in good health and protected from the inclemency of the weather ; against
the foe they must protect themselves, but their health
is a matter for which the State must provide. Hence
one sees the Turk better clothed than armed. He is
particularly afraid of the cold, against which, even in
the summer, he guards himself by wearing three garments, of which the innermost—call it shirt or what
you will—is woven of coarse thread and provides

much warmth. As a further protection against cold and rain tents are always carried, in which each man is given just enough space to lie down, so that one tent holds twenty-five or thirty Janissaries. The material for the garments to which I have referred is provided at the public expense. To prevent any disputes or suspicion of favour, it is distributed in the following manner. The soldiers are summoned by companies in the darkness to a place chosen for the purpose—the balloting station or whatever name you like to give it—where are laid out ready as many portions of cloth as there are soldiers in the company ; they enter and take whatever chance offers them in the darkness, and they can only ascribe it to chance whether they get a good or a bad piece of cloth. For the same reason their pay is not counted out to them but weighed, so that no one can complain that he has received light or chipped coins. Also their pay is given them not on the day on which it falls due but on the day previous.

The armour which is carried is chiefly for the use of the household cavalry, for the Janissaries are lightly armed and do not usually fight at close quarters, but use muskets. When the enemy is at hand and a battle is expected, the armour is brought out, but it consists mostly of old pieces picked up in various battlefields, the spoil of former victories. These are distributed to the household cavalry, who are otherwise protected by only a light shield. You can imagine how badly the armour, thus hurriedly given out, fits its wearers. One man's breastplate is too small, another's helmet is too large, another's coat of mail is too heavy for him to bear. There is something wrong everywhere ; but

they bear it with equanimity and think that only
a coward finds fault with his arms, and vow to dis-
tinguish themselves in the fight, whatever their equipment may be ; such is the confidence inspired by
repeated victories and constant experience of warfare.
Hence also they do not hesitate to re-enlist a veteran
infantryman in the cavalry, though he has never
fought on horseback, since they are convinced that one
who has warlike experience and long service will
acquit himself well in any kind of fighting. . . .

I will now return to the topic with which I dealt
before, namely, the indulgence which the Turks show
towards every kind of animal. The dog is regarded
by them as a foul and unclean animal, and they therefore exclude it from their houses ; its place there is
taken by the cat, which they regard as a much more
moral animal and apparently endowed with some
degree of modesty and propriety. In support of this
attitude towards the cat they quote the example of
Mahomet their lawgiver, who was so devoted to his
cat that, when it had fallen asleep on his sleeve while
he was reading and the hour of prayer called him to
his religious duties, he preferred to cut away his sleeve
rather than disturb the cat's slumbers. Although they
have this feeling about dogs, which are public property and have no masters and act as watchers over
quarters and districts rather than any particular
houses, and live on the refuse which is thrown out
into the streets, yet, if there is a bitch with puppies
in the neighbourhood, they go to her and make a heap
of bones and scraps of porridge and bread, and regard
such action as entirely pious. When I accuse them of
giving to a brute beast what I am inclined to think

they would not bestow on a rational being of their
own kind and certainly not on a Christian, their reply
is that reason has been given to man by God, a noble
instrument for every purpose, but that man abuses
this gift, and so any misfortune which befalls him is
due to his own fault and, therefore, he deserves less
pity ; on the other hand, God has bestowed upon the
brutes nothing except certain natural impulses and
appetites, which they cannot but follow, and, therefore, they are deserving of human help and pity. For
this reason they are enraged if any animal is put to
death by torture and any pleasure is taken in mutilat-
ing it. I can illustrate this by what happened lately
to a Venetian goldsmith. He used to take delight in
capturing birds, and had caught amongst the rest a
creature the size of a cuckoo and of much the same
colour, but with so huge and wide a throat, though its
beak was small, that, when it was forced open, it
gaped so wide that it could contain a large human fist.
The man, who was something of a joker, struck by
the strangeness of this, fastened the bird with wings
outstretched over the entrance to his house, with its
jaws held open with a piece of wood, so as to make it
gape. The Turks, who passed that way in large
numbers, stopped and looked up at it ; but when they
saw that the bird was moving and alive, they were
stirred to compassion, and exclaimed that it was
a crime thus to torture a harmless bird. They summoned the goldsmith from his house and seized him
by the scruff of the neck and haled him before the
judge who tries capital charges, and he was on the
point of receiving a good thrashing when a messenger
arrived from the Venetian Baily (n), the official who

administers justice to the inhabitants of Venetian nationality, and demanded that he should be handed over to him. The judge was kind hearted and well disposed, but the request was only granted with difficulty amid the protests of the other Turks. Thus the man was saved (n). He often used to visit me, and I was much amused when he told me the whole story and described how frightened he was. He also brought the bird for me to see ; I have already described its appearance, and it is said to fly at night and to suck cows' udders. I imagine that it is identical with the goat-sucker of the ancients. Such is the attitude of the Turks towards every kind of animal, and particularly towards birds.

Near our quarters is a tall plane tree, remarkable for its widespreading branches and the density of its foliage. Under it bird-catchers sometimes take their stand with a large number of little birds, and many people come and ransom the captives for a few coppers and then release them one by one from their hands. They generally fly up into the plane tree, where they cleanse themselves from the grime and dirt of their prison and spread their wings, chirruping the while. Then the Turks who have ransomed them say to one another : ' Listen to him congratulating himself and thanking me.'

' What,' you exclaim, ' are the Turks such Pythagoreans that in their eyes every animal is sacred and they never feed upon them ? ' By no means ; nay rather, they refrain from no flesh that is set before them whether boiled or roast. They declare that the sheep is born for the butcher's stall ; but they do not tolerate that any one should take pleasure in its agony and torture. The smaller birds, of whose notes the country and fields are full, some Turks can never be induced to kill or even keep shut up in cages, thinking it too great an interference with their liberty. But on this point there is a divergence of opinion. Some Turks certainly keep nightingales with sweet voices, and let them out on hire in the spring. I have seen men carrying about goldfinches trained to fly quite a long distance in search of a coin which was displayed to them from a window above. If the person who was holding the coin did not allow it to be wrenched from him, they would perch on his hand and accompany him from room to room, struggling all the time to seize the coin. As soon as they obtained it, remembering the way by which they had come, they would fly back to their master in the street, who recalled them by ringing a bell, and, on handing over the coin, received as a reward a few grains of hempseed. But enough of this subject, lest you should think that I am imitating Pliny or Aelian and want to write a Natural History.

I will now pass to another topic and tell you about the high standard of morality which obtains among the Turkish women. The Turks set greater store than any other nation on the chastity of their wives. Hence they keep them shut up at home, and so hide them that they hardly see the light of day. If they are obliged to go out, they send them forth so covered and wrapped up that they seem to passers-by to be mere ghosts and spectres. They themselves can look upon mankind through their linen or silken veils, but no part of their persons is exposed to man's gaze. The Turks are convinced that no woman who possesses the slightest attractions of beauty or youth can be seen by a man without exciting his desires and consequently being contaminated by his thoughts. Hence all women are kept in seclusion. Their brothers, it is true, are allowed to see them, but not their husbands' brothers. Men of the wealthier classes and higher ranks make it a condition, when they marry, that their wives shall never set foot outside their houses, and that no man or woman shall on any pretext whatever be admitted to visit them. This prohibition includes even their nearest relatives, except their fathers and mothers, who are allowed to visit their daughters at the Turkish Easter. If the wife is the daughter of a man of very high rank or has brought an unusually large dowry, the husband undertakes on his part not to keep any concubines but to be faithful to one wife. Otherwise, no law forbids a Turk to take as many concubines as he likes in addition to his lawful wife ; and there is no distinction between the children of wives and those of concubines, but both are held to possess the same rights. Concubines may be either purchased or acquired in war, and when they are tired of them there is nothing to prevent them sending them to the slave-market and selling them. They obtain their freedom, however, if they bear children. Advantage was taken of this privilege by Roxolana, Soleiman's wife, when she had borne him a son while she was still a slave. Having thus obtained her freedom and become her own mistress, she refused to have anything more to do with Soleiman, who was deeply in love with her, unless he made her his lawful wife, thus violating the custom of the Ottoman Sultans. The dowry is the only thing which distinguishes a lawful wife from a concubine ; for no slave has a dowry. A marriage-portion confers upon a woman the right to be mistress of her husband's household and gives her authority over all the other women. The husband, however, has the right to choose with whom he shall pass the night ; he intimates his wishes to his wife, who sends him the slave whom he has selected. The latter perhaps obeys with more alacrity than the other gives the order. One night a week is reserved for the wife, namely, Friday, which is their feast day, and she has a right to complain if her husband defrauds her of it. Of the other nights he may dispose as he pleases.

Divorces are granted amongst the Turks on many pretexts, which husbands can easily contrive. A divorced wife has her dowry restored to her, unless the separation has been due to some reproach against her. Wives have more difficulty in divorcing their husbands. Amongst the reasons for which it is granted are the failure on the part of the husband to supply his wife with the necessities of life and unnatural behaviour on his part. The wife then appears before the judge and testifies that she can no longer live with her husband ; when the judge inquires the reason, without giving any answer she takes off her shoe and turns it upside down. This indicates to the judge the treatment which she has received from her husband.

Men of position who possess large harems put them under the charge of eunuchs. . . . They also have baths in their houses for the use of themselves and their womenfolk ; the poorer classes use the public baths. They hate uncleanliness of the body as though it were a crime, and regard it as worse than impurity of the soul; hence their frequent ablutions. Since the majority of the women make use of the women's public baths, great numbers both of free women and of slaves congregate there, amongst whom are many girls of extraordinary beauty brought together by various chances from every quarter of the world. . . .

Roostem, when, after an interval of some days, I had been transacting some public business with him, began to treat me in a friendly way, which was rare with him, and eventually brought himself to ask me why I did not have myself initiated into their religion and become a partaker in the worship of the true God. He added that, if I were to do so, I might expect great honours and rewards from Soleiman. I answered that it was my fixed determination to abide in the religion in which I was born and which my master professed. ' So be it,' said Roostem, ' but what will become of your soul ? ' ' For my soul too ', I said, ' I have good hope.' Then, after reflecting for a moment, he said, ' Yes, you are right ; I cannot help thinking that those who have lived holy and innocent lives on this earth will share eternal bliss, whatever religion they may have practised.' This heresy is held by some Turks, and indeed Roostem is considered as not too orthodox in all respects. The Turks consider it quite in accord with their religion and duty to make a single offer of communion in their rites and cult to a Christian who enjoys their good opinion, hoping thus, if possible, to save one who is destined for everlasting destruction ; and they regard such an offer as the greatest act of kindness that they can show.

I must now repeat another conversation which I had with Roostem, which will show you what a wide difference of religion exists between the Turks and Persians (*n*). He asked me once whether war was still going on between the Kings of Spain and France. When I replied in the affirmative, he said, ' What right have they to wage war against one another, when they are bound by religious ties ? ' ' The same right,' I replied, ' as you have to go to war with the Persians ; there are cities, provinces, and kingdoms, about which they are at quarrel and have recourse to arms.' ' The cases are not parallel,' replied Roostem, ' I assure you that we abhor the Persians and regard them as more unholy than we regard you Christians.'

[Busbecq next gives an account of the campaigns of Ali Pasha in Hungary.]

In Croatia, too, and the neighbouring districts various raids have taken place from both sides of the frontier, and both parties have paid the penalty for excessive indolence and carelessness, and for excessive daring. I will quote an example, which gave me matter for rejoicing and will, I am sure, be pleasant hearing to you. . . . News had been brought from that part of the world to Roostem that a certain Turk, whom he praised very highly and declared to be a kinsman of his own, had suddenly put in an appearance with an armed force as a highly inconvenient guest at a wedding which some Christians were celebrating. They imagined themselves quite safe, for they lived in a remote district and had no idea that there were Turks anywhere near. The raiders caused a general confusion, killed a number of men, and carried off several persons, including the unhappy bridegroom and his intended bride. Roostem was delighted at the news and inflicted upon every one a boastful account of his kinsman's wonderful generalship. Up to this point the story provides food for commiseration rather than congratulation ; such events are the tragic sport of cruel fate. But vengeance was hard at hand to change Roostem's laughter to tears and grief. Not long after, a Dalmatian horseman arrived from the same district hot-footed (he was one of those men whom the Turks call ' Delli ', or madmen, from their excessive and stupid recklessness), and announced a serious reverse and defeat. Several Sanjak-beys and other garrison-commanders had joined forces and made a raid into the enemy's country. Sweeping over many miles of territory they had laid it waste and carried off much spoil ; but not knowing when to stop, they had at last fallen in with a force of Christians, mounted and armed with muskets, who had scattered them and put them to flight with great slaughter. They had to mourn the loss of many men, including Achilles, Roostem's relative, whose praises he had lately so loudly celebrated. Overwhelmed by the sad news, Roostem could not restrain his tears, and his grief for his friend's death was a well-deserved punishment for his former empty boasting. Now listen to the sequel, which is quite as entertaining. When the Dalmatian horseman, who, as I have said, brought the news of the disaster, was afterwards asked by the Pashas at the Divan, ' How many of you were there ? ' he replied, ' More than 2,500.' The Pashas then proceeded to ask, ' Well, what was the number of the Christians ? ' He answered that he thought they were not more than 500, unless, as he suspected, some of them had hidden themselves in ambush ; but certainly not more took part in the fight. At this the Pashas

expressed their anger that he was not more ashamed
that a regular force of Mussulmans (as they call the
men of their religion), picked warriors who had been
thought worthy of being supported by Soleiman and
had eaten of his bread, should have been scattered by
so small a band of Christians. The messenger, thereupon, by no means abashed, replied, ' I do not think
you understand the matter aright ; did I not tell you
that our men were overcome by the might of muskets ?
It was the fire that routed us, not the valour of our
foes. Very different, by my faith, would have been
the issue of the fight, if they had faced us with genuine
courage ; instead of that, they summoned fire to their
aid. It was the might of fire that overcame us, we
admit it—fire, one of the elements, nay the fiercest
of them. How can any mortal strength contend with
it ? Does not everything yield to the fury of the elements ? ' When the Dalmatian uttered these high-
flown sentiments, scarcely any one present, in spite of
the sad tidings, could refrain from laughing.

This incident cheered me not a little, though I was
saddened by the recollection of the previous mis-
chance. It showed me that the Turk is afraid of the
small muskets, such as are used by horsemen. I am
told that the same is true also of the Persian ; and for
this reason some one advised Roostem, when he was
setting forth with the Sultan against the Persians, to
arm with muskets a squadron of two hundred cavalry
selected from among his retainers, in order to inspire
the enemy with terror and cause great slaughter. He
followed this advice, formed the squadron, armed them
with muskets, and had them trained in their use. But
they had scarcely completed half the journey before

the usefulness of the muskets began to be impaired. Every day some part would be broken or lost, and there were few who could repair them. Thus the majority of the muskets had become quite useless, and the men wished they had never brought the weapons. Also they offended the sense of cleanliness, on which the Turks set so much store ; they were seen going about with their hands all begrimed with soot, their uniforms dirty, and their clumsy powder-boxes and pouches hanging down, so that they became a laughing-stock to their comrades, who jeeringly called them apothecaries. So, since with this equipment they displeased both themselves and others, they came to Roostem and displayed their broken and useless muskets, and asked what profit they were likely to gain from them when they faced the enemy ; they begged him to relieve them of them and to restore to them their accustomed weapons. Roostem, after carefully considering the matter, saw no good reason for refusing their request ; and so, with his kind permission, they resumed their bows and arrows.

The mention which I made just now of fighting on the Hungarian frontier reminds me that I ought to explain the attitude of the Turks towards duelling, which is regarded in our eyes as a unique proof of the highest courage. In the district of Hungary adjoining our territory lived a Sanjak-Bey, named Arslan Bey, who was famous for his strength. No one could draw a bow more mightily, or plunge his sword more deeply, or inspire greater fear in the foe. But a rival had presented himself, Veli Bey, the Sanjak-Bey of a neighbouring district, who aspired to the same reputation. Their rivalry, which was perhaps increased by other circumstances, led to bitter hatred, plots, and bloodshed. On this account, or perhaps for other reasons with which I am not acquainted, Veli Bey was summoned to Constantinople. Anyhow, he arrived and was asked many questions by the Pashas at the Divan, and finally about his quarrel with Arslan Bey. (In Turkish Arslan means lion.) He described in detail the whole history of their feud, its causes and its progress and its final result ; and, to strengthen his case, added that he had been ambushed and wounded by Arslan Bey, though he had no need to resort to such devices if he had wished to show himself worthy of the name which he bore. He would himself, he said, never have refused to fight him, since he had frequently challenged him to single combat. This speech disgusted the Pashas, who exclaimed, ' Did you dare to challenge a comrade in arms to fight a duel ? Was there any lack of Christians for you to fight ? Both of you eat our Sultan's bread ; yet you were prepared to fight one another to the death. What right had you ? What precedent for such conduct ? Did you not know that, whichever of you fell, the loss would fall upon the Sultan ? ' With these words they ordered him to be led away to prison, where he pined away for many months, and has only just been released with great loss of reputation. Yet, amongst us, many men, who have never set eyes on an enemy of their country, enjoy a great fame and reputation because they have drawn their sword against a fellow citizen or companion-in-arms. What are you to do with a code of morals according to which vices take the place of virtues, and conduct which deserves punishment is accounted glorious and honourable ?

Since you want to hear all I have to tell you, I must not fail to give you an account of the visit of the King of the Colchians to this city. His kingdom lies on the banks of the river Phasis, in a corner of the Black Sea, not far from the Caucasus, and his name is Dadian. He is a man of dignified mien and huge stature, but, according to all reports, of a low grade of civilization. He arrived with a large but ragged retinue, in poor and worn-out clothing. The Colchians are now called Mingrelians by the Italians. They are one of the tribes who have their abode between the Caspian Gates (which the Turks called Demir Kapu, or ' Iron Gates ') and the Black and Caspian Seas, and are now called Georgians, either from the kind of Christianity which they profess, or (as is more pro-bable) because it was their ancient name. Other neighbouring tribes are the Albanians and Iberians. The reason of his arrival is uncertain ; some suspect that he was invited by the Turks, since the Colchians and the other peoples of that region might be of great assistance to the Turk in his war with the Persians, if they were on his side. A more probable pretext, which is commonly alleged, is that he has come to ask for the assistance of some vessels of war against his neighbours, the Iberians, and, if he can obtain it, would be willing to pay tribute to the Sultan. The Iberians slew his father, and the Colchians have for a long time felt a deep hatred towards them. On one occasion, however, a conference was held with a view to peace and reconciliation, and the Colchians and Iberians met in large numbers. This resulted in an amusing incident. The two parties began drinking against one another, and held a competition as to

which should have the credit of drinking the most,
in which the Colchians proved themselves inferior
and lay overcome by deep sleep.   The Iberians then
treacherously placed the worthy Dadian, asleep and
snoring, in a carriage and bore him away, as though
he had been captured in fair fight, and confined him
in a lofty tower.   To avenge this wrong and recover
their king, the Colchians collected an army of 30,000
men under the leadership of the wife of the captive
monarch, a woman of great spirit and skilled in riding
and wielding weapons.   The chief commanders were
armed with heavy, clumsy breastplates and had swords
and spears shod with iron ; there was also, you will
be surprised to hear, a band of musketeers.   The rest
of the host had no armour to protect them, and fought
with arrows or stakes with burnt points and large
wooden clubs, and rode on horses without saddles.
They had absolutely no order or discipline ; and so,
when this irregular army approached the place where
their king was imprisoned, they were terrified by the
explosion of a few cannon balls, and retired a whole mile
in hurried flight.   They then recovered their courage and
again advanced ; but were again thrown into confusion by
the cannon balls, and this happened several times.   However, Dadian, seeing help close at hand, tore up the sheets
which covered his bed into strips and let himself down
from a window by night and escaped to his own people,
an exploit which is still commemorated as a marvellous
achievement in the stories of the peoples of that part.

The whole district in which the Colchians live is
rich in produce of every kind, which grows practically
without cultivation, except wheat and barley, which, it
is supposed, would also abound if a little trouble were

taken. The inhabitants, however, prefer to be idle.
Millet is sown in a slovenly manner and comes up in
the greatest abundance, its yield being so plentiful
that one crop suffices for two years. To this they have
become accustomed and eat of it in abundance, and
desire no better corn. They produce plenty of quite
tolerable wine from vines planted at the foot of the very
tall trees. These vines, spreading among the branches
over which they are trained, are productive for a long
period. Of wax and honey they have abundance from
the wild bees that produce them in the woods ; the
only trouble is to find out their haunts. The woods
also provide plenty of game, being full of pheasants
and partridges. A proof of the fertility of the soil is
provided by the melons, which not only have an excellent flavour but often grow to a length of three feet.

There is very little money among them ; very few
of them have ever seen a silver coin, still fewer a gold
coin, which scarcely any of them possess. I do not
know whether I should be wrong in saying that they
are lucky in thus lacking so strong a temptation to
crime ; however, if I mistake not, few of my countrymen would envy their happy condition, since no one
can grow rich amongst them. Silver is so highly
esteemed among them that, if any is brought into the
country through commerce with foreigners, as must
necessarily happen, it is all devoted to the use of their
churches, being melted down to make crosses and
chalices and other ecclesiastical ornaments. These
the King, when he thinks fit, melts down again on
the plea of public necessity, and converts to his own
purposes. Barter is the only form of commerce with
which they are acquainted ; every one brings to

market anything of which he has a superfluity and exchanges it with any one who requires it. They thus feel no need for money, the place of which is supplied by barter ; nay the taxes are paid to the King in kind, and these provide him liberally with all that his mode of life requires in the way of food, drink, and clothing, and for rewarding his household and those who serve him well. He has inexhaustible supplies both from the tithes and other royal dues, and also from the presents which are continually showered upon him, though he is quite as ready to bestow them as to accept them. His palace is a kind of public granary, packed with supplies of every description, out of which he bestows food on all. Any one who is in want or has fallen into poverty, and all those who have been disappointed by bad crops and the failure of their expectations, are fed from the royal stores.

There is a custom that all traders who put in at his shores should bestow some gift upon the King, who accepts it, whatever it may be, and invites the donors on landing to a feast. There is a vast building, at either end of which are the royal stables ; and in this the King's board is spread. It is very long, and the King himself sits at the top of the table and the rest of the guests at a little distance away. It is loaded with edibles of every kind, especially game, and wine is supplied in generous profusion ; indeed the deeper a man drinks, the more welcome he is as a guest. The Queen with the attendant women dines in the same dining-hall, but at a separate table, which, however, is not remarkable for dignity or decorum. The women are quite as free with their liquor as the men, and indulge in foolish gesticulations, laughter, nodding, and winking. Apparently if Jason were to visit the country again, he would find plenty of Medeas there (*n*). On rising from the table the King goes off hunting with his guests.

Everywhere in the woods of Mingrelia, under the shade of widespreading trees, you can see the common people reclining in groups and keeping holiday with wine and dance and song. They stretch strings on a staff or beam and strike them in regular time with a stick, and to this tune they sing love songs or the praises of their heroes, among whom, if what is said is true, the name of Roland frequently figures. How his name can have travelled so far I cannot guess, unless it came over with Godfrey de Bouillon (*n*). They tell many extraordinary tales about this Roland, even more absurd than are told by those who invent such fables among us. Where there is so much leisure and food is so abundant, the standard of morality is not high and chastity is rare. A husband introduces the visitor to his wife, or a brother to his sister, if he wishes to please him and enable him to pass the time pleasantly ; and they are so indifferent to what may result that they even consider it a matter for boasting if their wives prove attractive. The girls are no more strictly guarded or better looked after ; with the result that few are to be found who have reached womanhood and yet have remained chaste. There are many instances of girls of only ten years of age who are mothers. If you express your surprise and refuse to believe that such tiny creatures can have children, they show you an infant not much larger than a big frog—and this though as a race they are tall and of fine physique. They are so destitute of manners and politeness that, amongst other habits, they think that they are paying you a compliment and doing you an honour by making a kind of eructation in their throat. There is one accomplishment for which they show a real genius, namely, thieving ; and skill in theft is held in high esteem. The expert robber is looked upon as a great man, while he who is ignorant of the art is despised as a useless blockhead, hardly worthy to live. Indeed, such a person is looked upon as degenerate and hopeless by his brothers, and even by his father, and is given away, or sold cheap, to foreign traders to be carried off to some far country. An Italian traveller, who had visited the country, told me that a priest robbed him in a church of his knife ; though he perceived the theft, he pretended not to have done so, and then, in order that the priest might not imagine that he had not been detected, he presented him with the sheath, so that he might have something in which to keep the knife. When they enter a church, the presence of images of the Virgin Mother, St. Peter, St. Paul, and the other saints has but little interest for them ; but there is always one picture for which they look, that of St. George on horseback, and before this they prostrate themselves in adoration and imprint kisses all over it, not omitting even the horse's hoofs. St. George, they declare, was a man of might, a famous warrior, who often in single combat fought with the Evil Spirit on equal terms and was victorious, or at least left the field unbeaten.

I will now tell you something which you will read with astonishment. Oriental monarchs are not to be approached without gifts ; and so Dadian brought Soleiman a dish hollowed out of a ruby of such brilliance that its light would enable travellers at night to find their road as easily as at mid-day. ' I do not believe it,' you say. No more do I, and I do not ask you to believe it, but there are plenty of people who do. More sagacious people say that it is a small bowl of carbuncle or garnet, which was stolen from a son of the King of Persia, who was wrecked by a storm on the coast of Colchis, while trying to escape to Constantinople. Dadian also brought twenty white falcons, or some other kind of hawk which is said to be found in large numbers in Colchis. Such is the information which I wished to communicate to you about the Colchians and their customs.

As for your inquiries about my pursuits and manner of life in general, in answer to your question whether I ever leave my house, I do not generally do so unless I have dispatches from the Emperor for presentation to the Sultan, or instructions to protest against the ravages and malpractices of the Turkish garrisons. These occasions occur only twice or three times a year. If I wished from time to time to take a ride through the city with my custodian, permission would probably not be refused ; but I do not wish to put myself under an obligation, and I prefer that they should imagine that I think nothing of my close confinement. Indeed, what pleasure could it give me to parade before the eyes of Turks, who would rail at me or even hurl insults at me ? What I enjoy is the country and the fields, not the city—especially a city which is almost falling to pieces, and of whose former glory nothing remains except its splendid position. Constantinople, once the rival of Rome, is now laid low in wretched slavery. Who can look upon her without a feeling of pity and without thinking of the mutability of human affairs ? Besides, who knows whether the same fate may not be threatening our own land ?

So I stay at home and hold communion with those old friends, my books ; they are my companions and the joy of my life. In the interests of my health I have built a court, in which I play tennis before dinner. After dinner I practise with a Turkish bow, with which weapon this people is extraordinarily skilful. They begin to shoot at eight or even seven years of age and practise continuously for ten or twelve years. The result is that their arms become exceedingly strong, and they become so expert that no objective is too small for them to hit. The bows which they use are considerably stouter than ours, and, being shorter, are easier to handle ; they are not made of a single piece of wood but of sinews and ox horns fastened with glue and flax. A Turk after long practice can easily draw the string of even the stoutest bow right back to his ear ; yet any one, however strong, who was unaccustomed to this kind of bow, could not draw it sufficiently far to release a coin fixed between the bow and the string in the angle where the latter is attached to the notch. They aim with such certainty that in battle they can pierce a man's eye or any other part which is vulnerable. In the school where they are taught you can see them shoot with such skill that they can surround the white on the target, which is generally smaller than a thaler, with five or six arrows in such a manner that each arrow touches the edge of the white without actually breaking into it or encroaching on it. They generally stand about thirty feet from the target. They wear

on the thumb of the right hand rings of bone on which
the string rests when they pull it, while the arrow is
held in check by the knuckle of the joint of the left
thumb, which is extended—a very different method
from ours. The butt on which the target is marked
is raised about four feet from the ground, and consists
of sandy earth kept in place by boards. The Pashas
and men with large establishments make their slaves
practise archery at home, the more skilled acting as
instructors to the others. At their Easter Festival—
for the Turks, like us, have an Easter (n)—some of
them meet on the great plain above Pera, and there,
seated in a long line with their legs crossed like tailors
in our country, which is the usual mode of sitting in
Turkey, they first offer the prayers with which the
Turk prefaces all his undertakings, and then try who
can shoot the farthest. The competition is carried
out in a most orderly manner and in complete silence,
in spite of the huge crowd of spectators. The bows
which they use on this occasion are very short, and
therefore very stiff, and can only be bent by archers
who are very well trained. They also have special
arrows. The reward of victory is an embroidered
towel, such as we use for wiping our faces ; but the
glory of being victor is more esteemed than any prize.
The distances which they shoot are almost incredible.
The point reached by the arrow of the man who
shoots farthest in each year is marked by a stone.
Many stones are in existence which date from times
gone by and are considerably beyond those set up at
the present day ; these they believe to mark the points
reached by their forefathers, to whose strength and
skill in archery they confess that they cannot aspire.

In many streets of Constantinople and at cross-roads
there are shooting-grounds where not only boys and
young men but even men of more advanced years
congregate. An official is put in charge of the target
and looks after it, watering the butt every day, since
otherwise it would dry up and the arrows would not
stick in it ; for in the shooting-grounds they only use
blunt arrows. The custodian of the target is always
present and extracts the arrows from the earth, and
after cleaning them throws them back to the archers.
This entitles him to a fixed payment from every one,
which provides him with a livelihood. The front of
the target looks like a small door, which may perhaps
have given rise to the proverb about ' shooting against
the door ', which the Greeks applied to any one who
altogether missed the target. For I believe that the
Greeks formerly used the same kind of target, and
that the Turks adopted it from them. I know, of
course, that the use of the bow by the Turks is very
ancient, but there is no reason why, when they came
as conquerors to the Greek cities, they should not have
continued the use of the target and butt which they
found there. For no nation has shown less reluctance
to adopt the useful inventions of others ; for example,
they have appropriated to their own use large and
small cannons and many other of our discoveries. They
have, however, never been able to bring themselves to
print books and set up public clocks. They hold that
their scriptures, that is, their sacred books, would no
longer be scriptures if they were printed ; and if
they established public clocks, they think that the
authority of their muezzins and their ancient rites
would suffer diminution. In other matters they pay

great respect to the time-honoured customs of foreign nations, even to the detriment of their own religious scruples. This, however, is only true of the lower classes. Every one knows how far they are from sympathizing with the rites of the Christian Church. The Greek priests, however, have a custom of, as it were, opening the closed sea by blessing the waters at a fixed date in the spring, before which the sailors do not readily entrust themselves to the waves. This ceremony the Turks do not altogether disregard. And so, when their preparations for a voyage have been made, they come to the Greeks and ask whether the waters have been blessed ; and if they say that they have not been blessed, they put off their sailing, but, if they are told that the ceremony has been performed, they embark and set sail.

It was also a custom of the Greeks to open the cave in Lemnos, whence the earth called ' Goat's Seal ' (n) is derived, only on the 6th of August, the feast of the Transfiguration of our Lord. This custom the Turks observe even at the present day, and they wish the service to be performed to-day just as the Greek priest has always performed it there, while they themselves remain at a distance as spectators only of the rite. If you ask them why they do this, they reply that many customs have survived from antiquity the utility of which has been proved by long experience, though they do not know the reason ; the ancients, they say, knew and could see more than they can, and customs which they approved ought not to be wantonly disturbed. They prefer, they say, to preserve them rather than make any change which may be for the worse. This opinion, I am told, is so strong, that some

Turks have even wished to have their sons secretly baptized, because they declare that they have a suspicion that this rite must have some good effect, and cannot have been instituted without due reason.

There is one point about Turkish military manœuvres which I must not omit, namely, the old custom which goes back to the Parthians of pretending to flee on horseback and then shooting with their arms at the enemy when he rashly pursues. They practise the rapid execution of this device in the following manner. They fix a brazen ball on the top of a very high pole, or mast, erected on level ground, and urge their horses at full speed towards the mast; and then, when they have almost passed it, they suddenly turn round and, leaning back, discharge an arrow at the ball, while the horse continues its course. By frequent practice they become able without any difficulty to hit their enemy unawares by shooting backwards as they fly.

But it is time for me to return to my lodging, lest my keeper be wroth with me. All the time which remains over, after I have performed the exercises which I have described, is devoted to my books or to conversation with the citizens of Pera, who are of Genoese origin, and other friends. I cannot, however, do so without the consent of my cavasses. Their moods vary, and they have lucid intervals during which they show themselves more tractable. When these halcyon days occur, numbers of Ragusans, Florentines, Venetians, and sometimes Greeks and men of other nations visit me, either to greet me or for some other purpose. Strangers also call here from still more distant climes, whose conversation causes me great pleasure. A few months ago an amber

merchant from Dantzig arrived, who had bought up
the whole supply of this sap or pitch. As a large
quantity of amber is exported to Turkey, he was
anxious to know to what use it was put and whether
it was exported again to still more distant lands. He
finally discovered that it was sent to Persia, where it
is highly valued, being used for ornamenting rooms,
cabinets, and shrines. He presented me with a barrel
of what they call Juppenbier (spruce-beer), which is
certainly excellent. I was much amused by my Greek
and Italian guests, who, being quite unaccustomed to
such liquor, did not know what to call it. At last,
hearing from me that it was conducive to good health
and looking upon it as a kind of medicine, they called
it syrup; and as they continually asked for 'another
dose', so that they might try the flavour again and
again, they drank up my barrel at a single meal.

I sometimes have such easy-going cavasses—for
they are changed from time to time—that they would
not even object to my going out, if I wished to go, and
actually suggest that I should do so. But, as I have
said, I am in the habit of refusing their suggestions,
so that they may not imagine that it is in their power
either to gratify or to annoy me. I excuse myself
with the jesting remark that I have been so long in
the house that I have become part of its structure and
cannot be torn from it without the risk of its falling
in ruins; I will go forth once and for all, when I am
allowed to return to my native land. I am glad that
my household enjoys liberty, so that they may bear
with their long exile with greater equanimity. The
only annoyance is that quarrels often arise with
drunken Turks whom they meet, especially if the

Janissaries are not with them ; and even if they are
there they cannot always prevent blows being given
and received. It is a nuisance to me to be obliged to
defend my people from the accusations which are
brought against them ; but the cavasses save me from
a good deal of trouble by continually insisting on keeping the gates closed. I will give you a recent example
of the result of this practice. Philippo Baldi, an Italian,
a man of sixty years, recently arrived on a mission to
me from the Emperor. He had travelled too fast for
a man of such an age, with the result that he fell ill.
The doctor had ordered that he should have a lotion ;
but when the apothecary brought it the cavasse refused him admittance and would not allow him to take
the medicine to the sick man, and behaved in a most
brutal manner. The cavasse who was in attendance
on me at the moment had for a long time behaved
with courtesy and kindness towards us, but on this
occasion he seemed to become ferocious all of a sudden
and showed a savagery which was quite intolerable.
He actually threatened my would-be visitors with
blows from his stick. This roused my ire, and I determined to show him that his silly, puerile threats were
a mere waste of energy. So I posted one of my men
on the inside of the door with orders to keep it bolted
and not to open it to any one except by my orders.
The cavasse arrived in the morning to open the door
as usual, but, as the key produced no effect, he discovered that it was bolted on the inside. So he called
to my man, whom he could see through the chinks
where the doors met, and told him to let him in. My
man refused ; whereat the cavasse flew into a temper
and began to curse and swear. Then my servant

replied, ' You can babble as much as you like, but
you won't be allowed in here, or any of your people.
Why should I open the door for you, if you won't open
it for us ? You shut us in ; so we will shut you out.
You may lock the door from the outside as much as
you like ; I will take care that it is bolted from the
inside.' ' Did the ambassador order this ? ' asked the
cavasse. ' Yes.' ' Well, at any rate let me put my
horse in the stable.' ' No, I won't.' ' Well, then,
supply me with some hay and fodder.' ' There is
plenty in the neighbourhood for you to buy.' It was
my custom to invite this cavasse to my table or else
send him food from it ; on this occasion, however, for
a change, he remained outside and missed his meal,
while his horse was tethered to a neighbouring plane
tree. The Pashas and many high dignitaries pass this
way on their return home from the Palace. Seeing
the cavasse's horse, which they recognized by its
trappings, munching its hay at the foot of the plane
tree, they asked why it was there and not, as usual, in
the stable. The cavasse then told them what was the
matter, and that, as he shut us in, so we were shutting
him out, and his horse as well, and that he was not
being supplied with food or his horse with forage
The story, which was repeated to the other Pashas,
caused considerable amusement, and no doubt remained any longer that they were gaining nothing by
keeping me locked up, and that such petty annoyances
only incurred my contempt. Not long after, this
cavasse was removed and our confinement began to
be less strict.

The incident was referred to a few days later by
Roostem in a manner which is worth recording. An

aged man who had a great reputation for piety and
sanctity came to visit Roostem, and, among other
remarks, asked him—since the quarrel between the
Sultan's sons was so notorious and serious disturbances were threatening and indeed were on the point
of breaking out—why did he not conclude peace with
the Emperor and free Soleiman from anxiety from that
quarter ? Roostem replied that nothing was more
desirable, but how could it be brought about ? He
could not possibly concede the demands which I made,
and I refused to accept what he offered. ' And he
refuses,' he added, ' to give way to compulsion. Have
I not done all I can to make him accept my conditions ? I have kept him a prisoner for some years ;
I annoy him in countless ways, and I treat him roughly.
But what is the good ? He has hardened his heart to
everything. We are careful to keep him in the strictest
confinement ; he actually locks himself in by bolting
the doors. My trouble is all in vain. Any one else,
I am sure, would long ago have become converted to
our religion, in order to get rid of these annoyances ;
but he takes no notice.' This story was related to me
by persons who were present when the conversation
took place.

The Turks are prone to suspicion and have conceived an idea that the ambassadors of Christian
princes bring different sets of instructions, which they
produce in turn to suit the circumstances and the needs
of the moment, trying at first, if possible, to come to
an agreement on the most favourable terms, and then,
if they are unsuccessful, gradually agreeing to more
onerous conditions. For this reason the Turks think
it necessary to intimidate them, threatening them with

war or else treating them practically as prisoners and annoying them in every possible way, so that their sufferings may make them produce sooner the instructions which they have been ordered to reserve till the last possible moment.

[Busbecq then tells the story of a Venetian ambassador who brought a double set of instructions.]

On the arrival here of Baldi, whom I have mentioned, his advanced years made the Turks suspect that he had brought fresh instructions, in accordance with which we would allow ourselves to be bound by less favourable conditions of peace. They were afraid that, knowing the domestic anxieties of the country, I should misrepresent these new terms. They, therefore, thought it necessary to act with greater severity towards me, in order the more quickly and surely to extort the fresh conditions from me. With the same purpose in view, Roostem conceived the idea of threatening me with war by means of a jest. What do you think this was ? He sent me a very large melon of the kind which we call ' anguries ' and the Germans call *Wasserplutzer*. The water-melons which grow at Constantinople are extraordinarily pleasant to the taste and have red seeds inside them. They are called Rhodian melons, because they came originally from Rhodes, and are much eaten for quenching the thirst in very hot weather. A melon of this kind was sent me by Roostem through an interpreter on a very hot day, with a message expressing a hope that I should eat a fruit which was so seasonable and unrivalled for counteracting the heat ; he added that he was informed that there were quantities of this fruit at Buda and Belgrade of an even larger size—meaning cannon balls. I sent back a message of thanks for his gift, which, I said, I should consume with pleasure, adding that I was not surprised at his remark about Buda and Belgrade ; for this kind of fruit was also to be found in equally great abundance at Vienna. My answer was designed to show Roostem that I had perceived the point of his joke.

[Busbecq next relates the story of the quarrels of the Sultan's sons, Bajazet and Selim, which resulted in open hostilities and culminated in the defeat of Bajazet at the battle of Koniah (May 1559). Soleiman then crossed over into Asia Minor, in order, by his presence, to give moral support to Selim.]

When it became known that Soleiman was on the point of crossing over into Asia and the day of his journey was fixed, I announced to my cavasse that I wished to witness the Sultan's departure, and bade him come early that morning and open the gates for me, as he took the keys away with him each evening. He graciously promised to do so ; so I instructed the Janissaries and my interpreters to hire a room for me overlooking the road by which the Sultan was to depart. This order was carried out. The day arrived, and I was awake before dawn and waiting at the gates for the cavasse to let me out. I waited and waited, but he did not come ; so I sent various people to summon him, first the Janissaries, who used to sleep at the gates, and then my interpreters, who were waiting outside to be admitted. I gave all these orders through the chinks in the double doors, which were old and dilapidated. The cavasse kept on inventing different excuses for his delay, at one time saying that he was just coming, at another that he had some business to which he must attend. Meanwhile, time was passing, and at last I could hear the volleys of fire-arms, with which the Janissaries greet the Sultan as he mounts his charger. At this my temper was roused, for I saw that I was being tricked. Even the Janissaries were moved by my annoyance and just indignation ; so they suggested that, if my people within pushed with all their might and they themselves assisted from outside, the doors, which were old and weak, could be dislodged, so that the bolts would burst and a way be opened. I approved of the plan, and the doors gave way before our violent pressure. We rushed to the house where I had ordered the room to be hired. The cavasse had meant to prevent my coming. He was not really a bad fellow ; but when he had reported my wishes to the Pashas, they had not liked the idea that their master should be seen by a Christian at the head of the small army which he was leading against his son. They therefore told him to put me off by polite promises until the Sultan had embarked, and then invent some story or other to clear himself. But his wiles recoiled on his own head. When we reached the house, we found it closed, so that it was as difficult for us to get in there as it had been to get out of our own house a moment before. When no one answered our knocking, the Janissaries again came forward and offered, if I would take the responsibility, to break open the door or else climb in by a window and let me in. I forbade them to burst the door, but made no objection to their entering by the window. More quickly than I can describe it, they had made good their offer, and were inside the house and unbarred the door. On going upstairs I found the place full of Jews—a regular synagogue. They were astonished that I had been able to enter through closed doors. When they understood what had happened, an elderly lady, rather well dressed, came forward, and, in Spanish, remonstrated with me for my violence and the damage which I had done to the house. I replied that the bargain had not been kept, and that that was the reason of my breaking in ; and I protested that I ought not to have been thus tricked. She refused, however, to accept my explanation ; and there was no time for further discussion.

A window was allotted to me at the back of the house, looking out upon the street by which the Sultan was to leave the city. I was delighted with the view of the departure of this splendid army. The Ghourebas and Ouloufedjis rode in pairs, the Silihdars and Spahis in single file. These are the names given to the household cavalry, each forming a separate body and having its own quarters. Their total number is said to be about 6,000 men. There was also a vast number of the household slaves of the Sultan himself and of the Pashas and the other high officials.

The Turkish horseman presents a very elegant spectacle, mounted on a horse of Cappadocian or Syrian or some other good breed, with trappings and horse-cloths of silver spangled with gold and precious stones. He is resplendent in raiment of cloth of gold and silver, or else of silk or satin, or at any rate of the finest scarlet, or violet, or dark green cloth. At either side is a fine sheath, one to hold the bow, the other full of bright-coloured arrows, both of wonderful Babylonian workmanship, as also is the ornamented shield which is attached to the left arm and which is only suited

to ward off arrows and the blows dealt by a club or
sword. His right hand is encumbered by a light spear,
usually painted green, unless he prefers to keep that
hand free ; and he is girt with a scimitar studded
with gems, while a steel club hangs from his horse-
cloth or saddle. ' Why so many weapons ? ' you will
ask. My answer is that he is practised in the use of
all of them. ' But how,' you ask, ' can any one use
both a bow and a spear ? Will he seize his bow only
when he has thrown or broken his spear ? '   No : he
keeps his spear in his possession as long as possible,
and, when circumstances demand the use of the bow
in its turn, he puts the spear, which is light and therefore easily handled, between the saddle and his thigh,
in such a position that the point projects a long way
behind and the pressure of the knee holds it firm as
long as he thinks fit. When circumstances make it
necessary for him to fight with the spear, he puts the
bow into the quiver or else fixes it across the shield
on his left arm. I do not propose, however, to spend
more words in explaining the skill in arms which they
have acquired by long practice in warfare and continual exercise. On their heads they wear turbans
made of the whitest and finest cotton stuff, in the
middle of which rises a fluted peak of purple silk.
This head-dress is often adorned with black feathers.

After the cavalry had passed, there followed a long
column of Janissaries, scarcely any of whom carried
any other arms except their muskets. Almost all wore
uniforms of the same shape and colour, so that you
could recognize them as the slaves or household of
the same master. There was nothing very striking in
their attire, which had no slits or eyelet-holes ; for

they declare that their clothes wear out quite enough
without their making cuts in them themselves. The
only ornaments in which they indulge are plumes and
crests and the like, and here they let their fancy run
riot, particularly the veterans who brought up the rear.
The plumes which they insert in their frontlets give
the appearance of a moving forest. Behind them
followed their captains and colonels, each with their
distinguishing marks of rank. Last came their commander-in-chief, riding by himself. Next followed
the chief officials, including the Pashas ; then the
infantry forming the royal bodyguard in their special
uniform and equipment, and carrying their bows, for
they are all archers. Next came the Sultan's own
chargers, remarkable for their fine appearance and
trappings, led by grooms. The Sultan himself was
mounted on a splendid horse. His expression was
severe and frowning, and he was obviously in an angry
mood. Behind him were three young pages, one
carrying a flask of water, another a cloak, and the
third a casket. They were followed by several eunuchs
of the bedchamber. The rear of the procession was
formed by a squadron of about two hundred horsemen.

Having thoroughly enjoyed the spectacle, it only
remained for me to placate my hostess ; for I heard
a remark that the woman who had spoken to me in
Spanish on my arrival was a friend of Roostem's wife,
and I was afraid lest some rumour about me should
be carried to his house, which might make it appear
that I had acted discourteously. I therefore summoned my hostess and urged that she ought to have
remembered our agreement and not have shut the
door against me, after having agreed for a fixed pay-

ment to keep it open. However, apart from any questions of her deserts, I expressed my intention of carrying out my part of the bargain, though she had failed to keep her word, and of paying her what I had promised and something more as well. Having promised seven gold pieces, I asked her to accept ten, so that she might not regret my entry into her house. When she found more gold in her hand than she had expected, she suddenly changed her mind, and, bursting into compliments and thanks, converted the whole of her Jewish congregation to the same attitude towards me. The lady whom I have mentioned as the friend of Roostem's wife heartily supported her and joined in the chorus, thanking me warmly in her name. Cretan wine and some dessert were produced and pressed upon me ; however, I refused them and made the best of my way home, followed by the good wishes of all the Jewish tribe, meditating as I went a fresh discussion with my cavasse about my having broken my way out during his absence. I discovered him seated in deep depression in the vestibule. He began a long complaint, to the effect that I ought not to have gone out without his consent or have burst the door, and that my action was a breach of the law of nations, and so on. I briefly replied that, if he had chosen to come in proper time, as he had undertaken to do, there would have been no need for me to break my way out ; his violation of his promise, in his desire to play a trick upon me, had been the cause of what happened. Finally, I asked him whether they regarded me as an ambassador or as a prisoner. ' As an ambassador,' he replied. ' If you regard me as a prisoner,' I said, ' it is useless for me to be employed to make peace, for a prisoner is not a free agent. If, however, you regard me, as you say, as an ambassador, why, being an ambassador, do I not enjoy liberty, and why am I prevented from leaving my house when I wish to do so ? Prisoners are kept shut up, but not ambassadors. All nations allow ambassadors their freedom ; it is here that the law of nations comes in.' He must understand, I went on, that he was in attendance on me neither as a gaoler nor as a constable, but, as he had himself often insisted, to aid me by his services and to take care that no injury was committed against me or my servants. He then turned to the Janissaries and began to quarrel with them for having given me advice and helped my men to open the gates. They denied that I had needed any advice from them, and declared that they had merely obeyed me when I told them to open the gates, and that—as indeed had happened—very little effort had been required, for the doors had yielded to gentle pressure and nothing had been broken or smashed. Thus, willy-nilly, the cavasse was appeased, and nothing more was said about the matter.

A few days later I was myself summoned to cross the sea. The Turks thought it advisable in their own interests that I should put in an appearance in their camp and be courteously treated as the representative of a friendly sovereign. An abode was, therefore, assigned to me in a village near the camp, and I was very comfortably lodged. The Turks were in tents in the plains hard by. Here I lived for three months and had a good opportunity of visiting their camp and acquainting myself pretty well with their system of discipline. You would, therefore, have some cause of complaint if I did not give you some details on this subject. Putting on a dress of the kind usually worn by Christians in that district, I used to wander about everywhere, unrecognized, with one or two companions. The first thing that I noticed was that the soldiers of each unit were strictly confined to their own quarters. Any one who knows the conditions which obtain in our own camps will find difficulty in believing it, but the fact remains that everywhere there was complete silence and tranquillity, and an entire absence of quarrelling and acts of violence of any kind, and not even any shouting or merrymaking due to high spirits or drunkenness. Moreover, there was the utmost cleanliness, no dungheaps or rubbish, nothing to offend the eyes or nose, everything of this kind being either buried by the Turks or else removed from sight. The men themselves dig a pit in the ground with their mattocks and bury all excrement, and so keep the whole camp scrupulously clean. Moreover, you never see any drinking or revelry or any kind of gambling, which is such a serious vice amongst our soldiers, and so the Turks know nothing of the losses caused by cards and dice. . . .

I asked to be conducted to the slaughter-house, where they kill the cattle, so that I might see what meat there was for sale. I saw only four or five sheep at most, skinned and hanging there ; and yet this was the slaughter-house for the Janissaries, whose number in the camp amounted, I imagine, to four thousand at least. When I expressed my astonishment that so little meat was enough for so many men, they replied that very few of them take meat, and that the greater part of their rations was sent over from Constantinople. When I asked of what these rations consisted, a Janissary was pointed out to me who was seated there devouring off an earthenware or wooden trencher a mixture of turnip, onion, garlic, parsnip, and cucumber, seasoned with salt and vinegar, though it would perhaps be truer to say that it was hunger that was his chief sauce, for he could not have enjoyed his meal more if it had consisted of pheasants and partridges. They drink nothing but water, the common beverage of all living creatures ; and their frugal diet suits their health as well as it suits their purse.

I was all the more astonished at their behaviour because their fast (Ramazan), which corresponds to our Lent, was near at hand. Amongst us at this season in the best regulated cities, not to mention the camps, there is a universal din of games, dancing, singing, shouting, revelry, drunkenness, and delirium ; in fact, every one goes mad. There is, therefore, no wonder that the story has gained credence about the Turk who, having visited our country on state business as an ambassador at this period of the year, related on his return that the Christians at certain seasons become crazy and mad, but afterwards come to their senses and recover their sanity by being sprinkled with a kind of ash in their temples. It was quite remarkable, he said, to see the beneficial change brought about by this remedy ; you could hardly believe that they were the same persons. He meant Ash Wednesday and the festival which precedes it. Those who heard the story were all the more astonished, because the Turks possess various drugs which make men lose their wits, while they know of very few which enable them suddenly to recover them.

During the days immediately preceding the period of fast they make no change for the worse in their ordinary mode of life, and allow themselves no special indulgence in eating and good cheer and licence. On the contrary, they prepare themselves for abstinence by reducing their usual allowance of food, for fear that they may not be able to put up with the sudden change. The period of their fast is so fixed that it occurs fifteen days earlier each year, since their twelve lunar months do not make up a full year. Hence, if their fast is held in one year at the beginning of spring, six years later it will fall early in the summer. The period of fasting is confined to the space of one lunar month. The ordeal is most trying when it falls in the summer, because of the length of the days, for their observance consists of tasting nothing during the day, not even water ; nay, they even consider it wrong to wash out the mouth until the stars appear in the evening. The days which are longest and hottest and most dusty are naturally the most trying, especially for those who have to work and gain a livelihood by their own labour. They are allowed, however, to eat before the rising of the sun, when the stars have not yet been dimmed by its light (for the sun must not see any one eating during the whole period of the fast) ; and for this reason abstinence is easier to bear when it falls in the winter. In order that there may be no occasion for mistakes on cloudy days, the priests who are in charge of the mosques place candles in a kind of paper lantern on the pinnacles of the minarets, so that their light may show clearly that the time for eating has arrived. (It is from these minarets that the priests summon the people to prayer by loud cries, instead of the bells which we use). Seeing these lights, the people at last, after visiting the mosque and worshipping God in accordance with their rites, return and take a meal.

On summer days I remember seeing them returning in crowds from the mosque to an inn in the neighbourhood of my quarters, where snow, of which a continual supply is brought from Mount Olympus in Asia, was on sale, and asking for snow-water, which they drank, sitting cross-legged ; for their religion forbids them to eat or drink standing, if they can possibly avoid doing so. As I could not see distinctly in the twilight what they were doing in this position, I asked some of my friends who were learned in Turkish customs, and discovered that they were all of them swallowing great draughts of cold water in order to open the way for their food (for otherwise it would stick in their throats, which were dried by the heat and fasting), and also in order to stimulate their hunger by the coldness of the water. They have no prescribed diet during the fast, and their rules of abstinence do not prevent them from eating any food which is permitted at other times. If any illness should occur which prevents them from fasting, they may violate their fast, on condition, however, that they make up afterwards, when they have recovered their health, the number of days which they have lost owing to illness. Also when they are in the enemy's territory and anticipate immediate hostilities, they are warned to postpone their fast to another season, so that they may not engage in battle when they are weakened by hunger. If they show any hesitation in obeying this order, the Sultan himself takes food publicly at mid-

day in view of the army, so that all may be encouraged
by his example and do likewise. Just as during the
remainder of the year their religious scruples keep
them from tasting wine and they cannot do so without
committing a sin, so they are most particular in
observing this rule all through the period of fast, and
no one is to be found so wicked or abandoned as not to
shun even the odour of wine, much less drink it.

I often inquire why it was that Mahomet so sternly
forbade his followers to drink wine, and I remember
being told on one occasion the following story.
Mahomet once happened to be journeying to visit
a friend, and on the way stopped at mid-day at a
house at which a marriage feast was being celebrated,
in which he accepted an invitation to join. He was
immediately struck with admiration at the extreme
gaiety of the guests and their numerous demonstra-
tions of genuine goodwill, their grasping of hands,
embraces, and kisses. On inquiring from his host, he
learned that wine was the cause of this state of feeling ;
and so, on his departure, he called down a blessing on
this beverage, because it united mankind in such strong
bonds of affection. But on the following day, when
he entered the house on his return journey, he found
a very different state of affairs ; there were traces
everywhere of a fearful fight and the ground was red
with blood and strewn with parts of the human body,
here an arm and there a leg, and other broken limbs
were scattered about. On asking the cause of this
fearful state of affairs, he was informed that the
guests whom he had seen on the previous day had
become so intoxicated with wine that they had gone
mad and vented their rage in mutual slaughter and

caused a terrible massacre. It was on this account that Mahomet changed his opinion and laid a curse upon the use of wine and forbade it to his followers for ever.

Thus all is quiet, and silence reigns in their camp, especially at the season of their Lent, if I may so call it. Such is the powerful effect of their military discipline and the severe traditions handed down from their forefathers. There is no crime and no offence which the Turks leave unpunished. Their penalties are deprivation of office and rank, confiscation of property, flogging, and death. Flogging is the most frequent punishment, and from this not even the Janissaries are exempt, although they are not liable to the extreme penalty. Their lighter offences are punished by flogging, their more serious crimes by dismissal from the army or removal to another unit, a punishment which they regard as more serious than death itself, which is indeed the usual result of this sentence ; for being deprived of the badges of their corps, they are banished to distant garrisons on the farthest frontiers, where they live in contempt and ignominy ; or if the crime is so atrocious that a more impressive example must be made of the offender, an excuse is found for making away with him in the place of his exile. Such a man, however, dies not as a Janissary but as an ordinary soldier. The endurance of the Turks in bearing punishment is quite marvellous. They often receive more than a hundred strokes on their calves, the soles of their feet and their buttocks, and several cudgels of cornel-wood are often broken in the process, so that the executioner has frequently to say, ' Give me another one.' (n) Although remedies are promptly applied, it often happens that several pounds of mangled flesh have to be cut away from the parts which have been damaged. Yet, for all that, they are compelled to approach the official by whose orders they have been beaten, and kiss his hand and thank him and to pay a fixed sum to the executioner for each stripe. They regard the cudgel with which they have been beaten as a sacred thing, and have no hesitation in believing, as the Romans believed about their sacred shields, that the first cudgel fell from heaven. Moreover, that such suffering may not be without its consolation, they believe that the parts of the body to which the cudgel has been applied will after this life be free from the pains inflicted by the fires of Purgatory.

When I say that the camp was exempt from quarrels and tumults, I must except one disturbance which was caused by my own followers. Some of them had gone for a walk outside the camp along the shore, unaccompanied by Janissaries, and taking with them only some Italians who had professed Mahomedanism. These renegades enjoy, among other advantages, the chance to ransom prisoners. They go to the persons in whose possession such captives are, and pretend that they are their relatives or connexions, or at any rate their fellow countrymen. They declare themselves to be moved to pity by their misfortunes and beg their possessors to accept a sum of money and set them free or else make them over to themselves. The owners make no difficulty about granting this request ; whereas, if a Christian were to ask such a thing, they would refuse or only sell at a much higher price. My men having gone out, as I have already said, came

across some Janissaries who were washing themselves
by swimming in the sea with their heads loosely
wrapped round with pieces of linen instead of their
official head-dresses. The Janissaries began abusing
my men because they were Christians ; for the Turks
not only consider themselves at liberty to call Christians by opprobrious names and otherwise insult them,
but actually think that to do so is an act of piety,
because they may be induced through shame at the
insults heaped upon them to change for a better one
a religion which exposes them to such abuse. Being
thus provoked my men retaliated, and hurled their
insults back ; and finally blows succeeded words, the
Italians whom I have mentioned siding with my men.
The result of the fight was that the head-wrapper of
one of the Janissaries was, somehow or other, lost.
The Janissaries proceeded to their commander and,
having noticed which way my men went, denounced
them for the injury which they had caused. This
officer ordered them to summon my interpreter, who
had been present at the scuffle. They seized him as
he was sitting in front of the door, while I was actually
watching from the balcony above. I was most indignant that one of my men should be carried off
without my consent to a place from which it was
certain that he would not return without having
received a flogging (for by this time I had discovered
what was the matter), seeing that he was a Turk by
nationality. I hurried down and, laying my hand
upon him, ordered them to let him go. They did so,
but made all the more pressing complaints to their
commanding officer. He interrupted them with orders
that they should take more men with them and bring

before him the renegade Italians whom I have mentioned ; he warned them at the same time not to use
any force against me or the house in which I was
lodging. They therefore presented themselves again
with a great din and stood in the street demanding
the Italians with loud shouts and threats. The latter,
however, foreseeing what was likely to happen, had
already crossed over to Constantinople. So the
quarrel continued for a long time with much abuse
from both parties, until at last a cavasse who was
then in my service, an old man with one foot in the
grave, in great alarm, without my knowledge handed
them out some pieces of gold as the price of the lost
linen wrapper ; and so the dispute ended.

I have a special reason for telling you about this
incident, because it provided me with the opportunity
of learning from Roostem's own mouth the opinion
which the Sultan entertains about the Janissaries.
Hearing of the disturbance, he sent a man to me to
warn me—I use his own words—' to avoid any pretext of quarrel with the rascals.' ' Surely,' he said,
' I was well aware that it was a time of war, during
which they were masters to such an extent that not
even Soleiman himself could control them and was
actually afraid of personal harm at their hands.' And
these were no idle words from Roostem's lips, for he
was well aware of his master's uneasiness. There was
nothing which the Sultan so much dreaded as that
there might be some secret disaffection among the
Janissaries, which might break out when it was impossible to apply any remedy. His fears are not entirely
groundless. A professional standing army possesses
certain great advantages ; but it also has serious

drawbacks which must be counteracted by special precautions. The chief of these drawbacks is that the sovereign is kept in continual dread of a mutiny, and the soldiers have it in their power to transfer their allegiance to whomsoever they will. Striking illustrations of this might be quoted from history. There are, however, numerous precautions which may be taken against such an occurrence.

While I was at the camp, Albert de Wyss, a distinguished man of wide education, joined me. He is a native, if I mistake not, of Amersfort. He brought several presents for the Sultan from the Emperor— a number of gilt cups and a clock of ingenious workmanship, which had the form of a tower mounted on an elephant's back—also some money to be divided amongst the Pashas. These presents Soleiman desired that I should present to him in the camp in the sight of the army, as a fresh testimony of the friendship which he wished his subjects to believe to exist between himself and the Emperor, and as a proof that no military operations were impending on the part of the Christians.

After this digression I must return to Bajazet, who had betaken himself from the battlefield of Koniah to the seat of his government at Amasia, apparently determined to remain quiet if his father would allow him. He had yielded to his sense of grievance and his youthful ambition ; he seemed to intend henceforward to shape his behaviour so as to comply with his father's wishes. He did not cease to try and discover his father's attitude by letters and suitable intermediaries ; and indeed Soleiman showed himself not indisposed to a reconciliation. At first he made no objection to receiving his messengers, and read his letters and replied not unkindly to them ; so that a rumour went round the whole camp that the father and son were coming together again and that allowance would be made for the faults of Bajazet's youth, provided that for the future the dictates of duty were observed. As a matter of fact it was all a pretence of the clever old Sultan, acting on the advice of the Pashas, and he was waiting to entrap Bajazet and get him alive into his power. There was a fear lest, if he were reduced to despair, he would make with such speed for the territory of the King of Persia— his only possible refuge—that he would escape the watchfulness and vigilance of the local governors. Indeed Soleiman kept continually sending messengers to them warning them to guard the roads into Persia, so as to leave Bajazet no possible loophole of escape. Meanwhile, any one suspected of supporting and favouring Bajazet, if he fell into the Sultan's hands, was examined under torture and then secretly made away with. Among these were some friends whom Bajazet had sent to clear his guilt. . . .

Soleiman's plans, although they were kept strictly secret, were not unknown to Bajazet's friends, who from time to time warned him not to trust his father, and to beware of plots and to take an early opportunity of securing his own safety by any means in his power.

It often happens that a small incident leads to very serious consequences ; so, on this occasion, what is said to have induced Bajazet to act was the arrest in the camp of one of his spies, who was shortly afterwards publicly crucified by Soleiman's orders on the ground that he had been recruited by Bajazet after the latter had been forbidden to enroll any more troops. This, as it were, gave Bajazet the signal that he ought to form immediate plans of escape. Soleiman, who thought that he had secured his object of preventing his son's escape, and perhaps with the further object of deceiving him, ordered the army to return to Constantinople on the day following the Turkish Easter (Bairam).

On the very day of the feast, as soon as the ceremonies were concluded, Bajazet ordered his baggage to be packed at Amasia and began his ill-starred journey to Persia. He was well aware that he was going to the ancient foe of the house of Othman, but he was resolved to try and win any one's pity rather than fall into his father's hands. He was accompanied by all his followers except those incapable of bearing arms and the women and children, who were unequal to bearing the toils of the long journey. Among them was Bajazet's newly born son with his mother; he preferred to leave the innocent child to the mercy of his grandfather rather than let him share his calamitous and wretched flight. Soleiman ordered the child to be brought up at Broussa, being still uncertain what fate had in store for the father.

I should have returned to Constantinople on the day before the Turkish Easter (Bairam), had not my desire to see the ceremonies kept me in the camp. The Turks were about to celebrate the rites of this festival in a wide level plain in front of Soleiman's tents, and I felt doubtful whether such an opportunity of seeing them would ever occur again. I made arrangements that my attendants, by the promise of

a sum of money, should obtain a place, whence I could
see the spectacle, in the quarters of a Turkish soldier,
which stood on a mound immediately opposite and
overlooking Soleiman's tents. To this place I betook
myself at sunrise. I saw congregated in the plain
a mighty assembly of turbaned heads, listening amid
a deep silence to the words of the priest who led their
prayers. Each rank had its appointed position, and
the separate lines seemed to form hedges or walls in
the wide, open space in which they were arrayed. The
more distinguished bodies of men were posted nearer
the spot where the Sultan had taken up his position.
All the troops wore the same dazzling uniforms, their
head-dresses vying with snow in whiteness. The
different colours presented a variety which was most
pleasing to the eye. So motionless did they stand that
they seemed fixed or rooted in the ground. There
was no coughing, no clearing of the throat, not a word,
no turning of the head or backward glance. When
the priest pronounced the name of Mahomet, all
together bowed their head to their knees. When the
name of God was uttered, they all fell on their faces
to the ground in adoration and kissed the earth. The
Turks join in their religious rites with great reverence
and attention, for they imagine that, if they as much
as scratch their heads, the effect of their prayer is
destroyed. ' For,' they argue, ' if you have to converse with a Pasha, would you do so in anything but
a respectful attitude ? How much rather, therefore,
should you observe such a posture before God, who
so far surpasses all human greatness ? ' When the
prayers were finished, the close array was broken up
and began to mingle and surge over the plain and

inundate the whole of its surface. Presently those whose duty it was brought the Sultan's dinner ; when, lo and behold ! the Janissaries laid hands upon the dishes and seized all the food and ate it up amid great merriment and gaiety. This privilege is allowed by ancient custom as part of the festivity of the occasion, and the Sultan's wants were provided for from elsewhere. I returned to Constantinople much delighted by the spectacle.

There still remains a little more to tell you about Bajazet ; then I will release you, for you are perhaps as tired of reading as I am of writing. Bajazet, having, as I have told you, left Amasia with his troops in light marching order, travelled so quickly that he generally arrived before tidings had been received of his approach, and found that most of those who had been ordered to look out for him were not expecting him and were unprepared. . . . His departure was a severe shock to Soleiman, who was rightly convinced that he was making for Persia. He could scarcely be restrained from advancing with all the infantry and cavalry of the guard and making a demonstration against the Persians. His advisers, however, checked his rash impetuosity by pointing out the danger of treachery on the part of the army. . . .

Bajazet's force was not indeed a large one, but it was warlike and contained brave men ready to run any risk, whom the Persian King had every reason to fear. The latter was conscious that his dynasty had not been long established, and had based its claim to rule on the pretence of religion (*n*). Who could be certain that, among the many peoples over whom he ruled, there were not many who disliked the existing régime and would therefore prefer a change, for which the arrival of Bajazet provided the best possible opportunity ? At present, he reflected, he was himself at the mercy of Bajazet rather than Bajazet in his power ; this state of affairs must end and Bajazet be no longer treated as a guest but chained up like a wild beast. This could easily be achieved if his troops could be dispersed and he were seized when he had no longer the protection of his bodyguard, for he could not be defeated in open warfare without serious bloodshed. The Persians were enervated by a long peace and were not concentrated, while Bajazet's army was on the spot, ready to fight, and well trained.

The plan, therefore, of disbanding his troops being placed before Bajazet and the arguments in favour of this course set forth, he was unable to raise objections, although the arrangement gave rise to grave suspicions in the minds of the more prudent and foreseeing of his followers. Yet how could he refuse ? His position was desperate, and he had no other hope of safety ; his life was at the disposal and mercy of his host, and to doubt the latter's good faith might be ascribed to the most treacherous intentions. Bajazet's troops were therefore conducted in separate parties to various villages, never to see one another again, and quartered where the Persians thought fit. A few days later, when a suitable occasion arrived, they were surrounded in small detachments by superior forces and put to death. Their horses, arms, clothing, and other equipment were given as spoil to their murderers. At the same time Bajazet was seized at the King's very table and while enjoying his hospitality—a circumstance which, in the opinion of some people, aggravated the baseness of the deed—and thrown into chains. His children were also incarcerated.

I have now given you, in accordance with your request, all the news of Bajazet up to the present date. What is likely to happen in the future I do not think any one can easily conjecture. Various opinions are held. Some think that he will be allotted Babylonia, or some similar province on the frontier of the two kingdoms, to rule as Sanjak-bey. Others repose no confidence either in King Sagthama or in Soleiman, holding that all is over with Bajazet, who, they think, will be sent back here for punishment or else will perish miserably in prison. The Persian, they say, knew what he was doing when he used force against Bajazet, his object being to prevent a vigorous and high-spirited young man, who is a much better soldier than his brother, from succeeding his father on the throne and thereby causing much trouble to himself and his kingdom. It would suit his interests much better if Selim, who is naturally gluttonous and slothful, ascended the throne, since then there would be pro-mise of peace and lasting security. Hence the Persian will never let Bajazet escape alive out of his hands, but will rather put him to death in prison, plausibly accounting for the young man's death by saying that he perished of disappointment and inability to endure confinement. Anyhow, he can never hope that one whom he has injured so deeply will ever be his friend.

Thus opinions differ ; my own feeling is that, how-ever matters turn out, it will be an awkward business. I wish that it may be so ; for the fortunes of Bajazet and our interests are closely connected. The Turks will not readily turn their arms against us until they have settled his business. Moreover, they are now trying to press upon me, for transmission to my master, a letter and terms of peace of the purport of which I am ignorant, but which they wish me to believe are very nearly in agreement with his wishes. They do not observe the usual custom of giving me a copy, and this makes me suspect some deceit, and so I am refusing to send any dispatches to the Emperor without their contents being first made known to me. If, after providing me with a copy, they should yet deceive me, their imposture will be manifest and no blame will attach to me. I am resolved to persevere in this course and so relieve my master of the difficulty of replying to their quibbling dispatches ; for he will accept no terms of peace which are not fair. It may appear that to reject peace, on whatever terms it is offered, is to pave the way to hostilities ; but I consider it best to leave everything open and wait and see what the future will bring. Meanwhile, the blame for not forwarding the dispatches will rest on my head, and I think that I can easily exculpate myself if the result of Bajazet's affair does not correspond with the wishes of the Turkish authorities. In the other event, I shall have a rather more difficult task, but there is nothing which I cannot explain and smooth over by putting forward suitable excuses. The Turks do not usually show any lasting resentment against those who they see are striving to promote their master's interest as best they can. Another point in my favour is the Sultan's increasing age, which, in the opinion of the Pashas, requires rest and quiet, and should not be exposed without necessity to the toils of warfare. Burdens and vexations are likely to continue to be my lot, but they must be borne with equanimity, provided they are not being undertaken in vain.

I am sending you a book rather than a letter ; but if I am to be blamed, so also are you to no less a degree. It was you who set me to the task, and it is at your request that I undertook to carry it out. My willingness to obey is the only charge which can be made against me, and such behaviour on the part of a friend is generally commended. I am not without hopes, however, that you will not find it burdensome to read what I have taken so much pleasure in writing. After I had once begun to write, I took a delight in beguiling my imprisonment by letting my mind wander far away and converse with you as though we were face to face. All my many irrelevant and trifling remarks you will have to accept as the random talk which passes in the familiar conversation of friend with friend. The same licence has usually been extended to a letter as to a conversation ; just as no one expects accurate judgement or careful expression in familiar talk, so, too, no pedantic criticism ought to be applied to a letter. When chatting with a friend one says what first comes to one's lips, and the same liberty is permissible in writing an intimate letter ; to use greater circumspection would be to abandon the privileges of friendship. Monuments which are destined to adorn temples and porticoes and to be always in the public eye call for a perfection which is unnecessary in articles of domestic use intended for private dwellings. So my letters are quite unworthy of the public gaze ; they are merely written for you and the few friends to whom you may wish to show them ; they make no claim either to erudition or originality. If they win your approbation, that is to say, if you read them with pleasure, they will have attained their object. They might be written in better Latin and with greater elegance ; who denies it ? But what if it is the best I can do ? It is a question not of will but of capacity. Indeed, you can hardly expect good Latin at the present day from a Greek land (*n*), or elegance of style from such an utterly barbarous country as Turkey. Lastly, if you do not despise my present letter, I undertake that you shall receive a further instalment describing my adventures up to my return to Vienna, if indeed I ever do return ; anyhow, I intend to stop writing now and bore you no longer.   Farewell.

THE FOURTH LETTER

I WELCOME your congratulations on my safe return as another proof of your kindness of heart and the goodwill which you have always shown towards me. As for your Excellency's request for an account of the rest of my mission and the events which have occurred since my last letter and any amusing incidents which I have observed, I have not forgotten my promise. I am fully aware of the obligations which I have undertaken, and have no intention of breaking my word or of defrauding so accommodating a creditor as yourself. Here, then, is an account of all that has happened since I last wrote, whether trifling or amusing or serious—in fact, as before, everything that I can remember. I am afraid, however, that I shall begin on anything but a cheerful note.

My spirits had scarcely recovered from the news of Bajazet's disasters and imprisonment, when we were disturbed by further news equally unfavourable. We were expecting to hear the result of a Turkish naval expedition which had sailed to the island of Meninx, or Jerba (n), as it is now called, owing to the reports of Spanish successes in that region. On hearing that this island had been captured by the Christians and that they had added new fortifications to the ancient citadel and had garrisoned the place, Soleiman felt that, as lord of so mighty and so flourishing an empire, he could not put up with the affront. He had therefore resolved to send his fleet to the help of a nation so closely bound to him by the ties of a common religion,

and had appointed Piali Pasha as admiral in command
of the expedition. The ships were manned with a large
number of picked men, who, however, were not free
from anxiety and alarm at the distance of the journey
and the reputation of their enemies. The minds of
the Turks had been deeply impressed by their experience of Spanish bravery in the many wars, both in
recent and in former times, in which success had
brought glory to their arms. They remembered the
Emperor Charles ; they heard daily reports of King
Philip, who had inherited his father's valour as well as
his throne. So great was their apprehension that many
of them, thinking that they were bound on a desperate
adventure from which they might never return to
Constantinople, made their last will and testament
before setting out. The whole city was full of alarm,
and every one, whether he embarked or stayed at
home, was harassed by grave doubts as to how the
expedition might end.

The fleet, however, enjoyed favouring winds and
came upon our men unawares ; and its unexpected
arrival caused such a panic that they had neither the
courage to fight nor the presence of mind to escape.
A few galleys, it is true, which were cleared for action,
sought safety in flight ; the rest stuck fast, or broke
up in the shallow water, or were surrounded by the
enemy and sunk. The Duke of Medina, who was the
military commander, took refuge in the citadel together
with Giovanni Andrea Doria, the admiral of the fleet.
Under cover of the darkness they embarked in the
early watches of the night and succeeded in passing
unobserved through the enemy's guard-ships in a
rowing boat and reached Sicily.

Piali sent a galley to Constantinople to announce his
victory. This vessel, in order to emphasize the purport
of the news which it brought, trailed behind it in
the water a banner, which, according to the Turkish
account, was painted with a picture of our Saviour on
the cross. When it entered the harbour, the rumour
of the defeat of the Christians quickly spread through
the city, and the Turks congratulated one another on
their great victory. They also congregated in crowds
round my door and mockingly asked my people
whether they had had a brother or relation or friend
in the Spanish fleet ; for, if so, they would have the
pleasure of seeing them shortly. They were also
voluble in extravagant praise of their own valour and
scorn of our cowardice. ' What forces,' they asked,
' remained to oppose them, now that the Spaniard
was conquered ? ' My men, to their sorrow, had to
listen to these taunts. What had happened was God's
will and nothing could change it, so they had to endure
it. The only hope that sustained us was that the
citadel, which the Spaniards still held with a large
garrison, might hold out until the bad weather or some
accident should cause the enemy to raise the siege.
Stronger, however, than this hope was the fear that,
as usual, success would favour the victors rather than
the conquered. And so indeed it turned out ; for the
besieged, harassed by their lack of supplies and
especially of water, eventually surrendered the citadel
and their own persons. Don Alvaro de Sandé, who
was in command of the troops there, a man of great
courage and military reputation, when he saw that he
could hold out no longer, broke out of the citadel
with a few men and seized a small ship with the inten-

tion of crossing over to Sicily. His object was that
he might not sully the great prestige which he had
won in warfare, by the disgrace of a surrender, however necessary, and that the loss of the place might
be ascribed to any one but himself. The result of his
action was that the citadel fell into the enemy's hands ;
for the soldiers opened the gates, which it was useless
any longer to close to the enemy, in the hope of thus
gaining more lenient treatment. Don Juan de Castella
refused to leave the rampart entrusted to his care, and
fought, together with his brother, until he was wounded
and finally taken prisoner.

The citadel had been defended by the Spaniards
with great devotion for more than three months,
though almost every kind of necessary supply and,
what was still worse, all hope of relief had failed. In
that hot climate nothing causes so much suffering as
thirst. There was only one cistern, which, though it
was large and well filled with water, could not suffice
for so large a number. Consequently the water was
rationed, just enough being distributed to each man
to keep him alive. Most of the men increased their
portion by adding sea-water, which had been purified
of the great part of its salt by distillation—a timely
device which a skilful chemist had shown them. Not
all of them, however, possessed the necessary facilities,
and therefore many of them were to be seen stretched
on the ground on the point of death, with their mouths
agape and continually repeating a single word, ' water '.
If any one took pity on them and poured a little water
into their mouths, they revived and sat up and remained in that posture until the effect of the water
wore off, when they fell back again and eventually

expired from thirst. Many died in this manner every day in addition to those who perished fighting or from disease and the complete lack of medical stores in that desolate spot.

In September the victorious fleet returned to Constantinople with the prisoners, spoils, and captured vessels, a sight as joyful to the Turks as it was mournful and deplorable to us Christians. The first night it anchored at the rocks off Constantinople, so that it might enter the harbour by day with greater pomp and before a greater crowd of spectators. Soleiman had gone down to the colonnade adjoining the entrance to the harbour and forming a continuation of his garden, so that he might have a nearer view of the arrival of the fleet and of the Christian officers exhibited upon it. On the poop of the flag-ship were displayed Don Alvaro de Sandé and the admirals of the Neapolitan and Sicilian fleets, Don Berenguer de Requesens and Don Sancho de Leyva. The captured galleys were towed along, stripped of their oars and bulwarks and reduced to mere hulks, so that in this condition they might seem small, shapeless, and contemptible in comparison with the Turkish vessels.

Those who saw Soleiman's face on this occasion declare that they could not detect any traces of unusual elation. Certainly I myself, when I saw him two days later setting out to perform his religious duties, remarked that his expression of face was unaltered. His countenance was marked by the same sternness and sadness, so that you would almost have thought that the victory was no concern of his and that nothing new or unexpected had happened. So steeled was the old man's heart to accept whatever fortune might decree, so unflinching his mind, that he seemed to accept all the applause without emotion.

A few days later the prisoners were brought to the Palace. They were starving and half-dead ;. most of them could scarcely stand, many of them were collapsing through weakness and fainting, some were practically dying. They were made a laughing-stock, being forced to wear their armour back to front or at any rate put on in a ridiculous manner. The cries of the Turks were to be heard all round uttering insults and proclaiming themselves the masters of the whole world ; for, now that the Spaniards had been vanquished, what enemy remained whom they need fear ?

A Turkish officer of high rank, whom I knew well, had taken part in the expedition. Into this man's hand had fallen the chief, or royal, standard of the Neapolitan fleet, which displayed the arms of all the Spanish provinces supported by the imperial eagle. Learning that he intended to offer it as a present to Soleiman, I thought it my duty to take steps to prevent this and obtain it from him. I had no difficulty in getting possession of it by sending him a gift of two silk dresses. I thus prevented the glorious insignia of Charles V from remaining in the enemy's hands as a perpetual memorial of the defeat.

Amongst the prisoners, besides those whom I have mentioned, were two officers of high birth, Don Juan de Cardona, the son-in-law of Don Bellenguer, and Don Gaston, the son of the Duke of Medina. The latter, though still almost a boy, had held high rank in his father's army. Don Juan had cleverly contrived, by the promise of a large sum of money, to be left

behind at Chios, which is still in the hands of its
ancient inhabitants, the Genoese. Piali had been
tempted by the hopes of obtaining a large ransom to
secrete Gaston, a plot which nearly caused his own
ruin. For Soleiman, having somehow or other got
wind of this, was exceedingly annoyed and, at Roostem's instigation, made strenuous efforts to unearth
Gaston from his hiding-place, in order that he might
catch Piali red-handed and have a good pretext for
punishing him. But his trouble was all in vain, for
Gaston suddenly died, either from plague, as some
believe, or else, more probably, through the agency of
Piali, for fear that some evidence might come out
against him. At any rate, though the most careful
inquiries were made by his father's agents, the truth
could not be discovered. It is only too likely that
Piali made away with Gaston in the interests of his
own safety. Anyhow, he lived for a long time in great
fear and shunned the neighbourhood of Constantinople, wandering about with a few vessels among the
islands of the Aegean on various pretexts ; he avoided
any approach to his angry master's presence, which
he knew would be fatal to him ; for he was convinced
that he would be thrown into prison and obliged to
defend himself. Finally, however, Soleiman, softened
by the prayers of the chief eunuch of the bedchamber
and of his son Selim, extended to him his pardon in
words which it gives me pleasure to repeat : ' For
myself, I grant him pardon and impunity for the terrible
sin which he has committed ; but, this life ended, may
God, the just avenger of crime, inflict upon him the
penalty which he deserves.' So convinced was Soleiman that no crime is destined to go unpunished.

Don Juan de Cardona met with better fortune. Thanks to the efforts of the illustrious Adam de Dietrichstein, an Austrian baron, who had married his charming sister, he was allowed to return in safety to Spain after I had undertaken to stand surety for him.

When de Sandé was brought before the Divan, or assembly of Pashas, and was asked by Roostem, ' what had induced his master to attack the territory of another sovereign when he could not protect his own,' he replied that ' it was not for him to criticize ; his duty was to carry out the orders of his master as faithfully as he could, but fate had been against him.' He then kneeled down and intreated the Pashas to recommend Soleiman to spare him, saying that he had a wife and several children, for whose sake he begged them to save him. Roostem answered that his master was merciful and that he hoped to obtain the preservation of his life. Orders were therefore given to convey de Sandé to the castle of Caradenis, that is to say of the Black Sea (*n*). But soon after his departure he was recalled, the sole reason being that the chief eunuch of the bedchamber, whom I have already mentioned, and who had great influence with the Sultan, had not seen him and wished to do so. Those who saw him returning state that, though a man of intrepid courage, he came back in a state of terrible emotion, being afraid that his sentence had been reversed and that he was brought back for execution. The other captives of note were incarcerated in the town of Pera, or Galata, as it is sometimes called. Among them were Don Sancho de Leyva and his two natural sons, and Don Berenguer. Hearing of this and of the terrible privations under which they were suffering, I thought it my duty to relieve their distress. I therefore sent persons to visit them and express my condolences and promise them any help that I could give them. From that time onwards my house was always open to a whole tribe of prisoners, and I never ceased to perform such services towards them as lay within my power.

The Turks think that they have amply provided for the needs of their captives if they supply them with bread and water. They take no thought of the age of the individual prisoners, their habits of life, their health, or the season of the year, and deal out the same treatment to the healthy and to those who are sick or recovering from illness, to the robust and to the delicate, to the young and to the old. Thus a wide field was open to me for giving various kinds of assistance to their different necessities. A large number of the sick lay in a mosque at Pera, as the town is called which lies immediately opposite Byzantium across the bay. These men were regarded by the Turks as hopeless cases, as good as dead and buried. Many of them, either while actually ill or in the course of recovery, died from want of a suitable diet—a little soup or some dainty morsel to tempt their failing appetite and enable them gradually to recover their lost strength. Hearing of this, I arranged with a friend of mine who lived in Pera to buy several sheep each day and boil them in his house and distribute the broth to some and the meat to others of the prisoners, as the state of each man's disease or convalescence demanded. This was of benefit to not a few of them.

Such was my work for the sick; those who were well demanded help of another kind. My house was

thronged from early morning till evening by those
who sought my aid in their various troubles. Some,
who had been accustomed to a luxurious table, could
not stomach a daily diet of dry black bread, and required the means to purchase some kind of relish.
There were others whose digestions could not put up
with having nothing to drink but water, and needed
a little wine. Others had to sleep on the bare ground
and could not endure the cold at night ; these had to
be provided with blankets. Others needed cloaks or
shoes. Most numerous were those who asked for the
means to mitigate the cruelty of their masters or
gaolers and render them more amenable. The only
remedy for all these troubles was money, and for
this I was continually asked ; so that no day passed
on which I did not spend several pieces of gold.

All this, though troublesome, was endurable and
not likely to ruin me. A more serious problem
threatened me in the demands of those who wanted
to borrow larger sums or wished me to act as surety
for their ransom. Every one of them had some special
plea in support of his claims, and tried to make his
own case appear the most pressing. One man would
urge his high birth and connexions, or the distinctions
and high office held by his relatives ; another the com-
mission which he had held and his long years of service ; another the wealth which he possessed at home
and his ability to pay back a loan with promptitude.
Not a few proclaimed their personal valour and warlike exploits. In a word, all had some reason or other
for claiming my aid. When any question was raised
about their good faith and the likelihood of their
remembering to pay, they told me that I need have no

doubts ; for what, they said, could be more unjust than to fail to release from anxiety and pecuniary loss a man who had rendered them so great a service, to whom they owed their life and liberty, and who had snatched them from the very jaws of death ? It was indeed most distressing to hear such appeals as this : ' If I cannot have two hundred pieces of gold in ready money, I am a lost man ; I shall be sent over into Asia, or become a galley-slave, and be carried off I know not whither, with no hope of ever recovering my liberty or ever seeing my home again. There is a merchant who will provide a sufficient quantity of goods to raise this sum, if only you will act as surety.' This was generally all the security that they could offer ; but I could not but be moved by the consideration that what they said was true, namely, that most of them would certainly perish in various ways unless help was forthcoming, and there was no one on the spot who had better means than I had of assisting them, or upon whom they had a stronger claim.

I can hear you blame me and say that no one is to be trusted ; but, I ask you, could any one possibly imagine that a man would be so outrageously ungrateful after he has been rescued from such imminent peril, as not to pay back the price of his life ? Perhaps one or two are without, not the will, but the means to do so. If so, I must not mind ; a good action performed for a good man is never wholly lost. Most of them will certainly keep their word. . .

This defeat of the Christians at sea, following upon the disaster of Bajazet, made one very anxious lest the Turks should become more arrogant and therefore less accommodating in the terms of peace which they offered me. On the top of these public misfortunes there had come a private trouble—a plague which had attacked my household and carried off one of my most faithful servants and caused great alarm among the rest, owing to their fear of contagion. I will tell you more of this later on, after I have mentioned another lesser, but still serious, cause of anxiety which befell us.

The Sultan is becoming day by day more scrupulous in his religious observance, in a word, more super-stitious. He used to enjoy listening to a choir of boys who sang and played to him ; but this has been brought to an end by the intervention of some sibyl (that is to say, some old woman famous for her profession of sanctity), who declared that penalties awaited him in a future life, if he did not give up this entertainment. He was thus induced to break up and commit to the flames all the musical instruments, even though they were ornamented with fine work in gold and studded with precious stones. He used to eat off a service of silver plate, but some one found such fault with him for this that now he only uses earthenware

Next some one presented himself who could not tolerate the extensive drinking of wine in the city and stirred up the Sultan's scruples on this subject on the ground that he was scarcely observing the precepts of the Prophet. An edict was therefore passed for-bidding the importation of wine into Constantinople in the future, even though it was intended for Chris-tians and Jews. This edict closely concerned me and my people, since we were quite unaccustomed to drinking water only. For how could we obtain wine if its introduction within the walls were to be pro-

hibited ? Our continual pinings for home and the
prolonged uncertainty as to how our negotiations
would turn out was reducing our strength without
the further necessity of a change in our diet, which
could not be carried out without harm to the health
of many of us. I instructed my interpreters to plead
our cause persistently with the Pashas in the Divan
and to uphold our former rights. Opinions varied ;
some considered that we ought to be content with
water. What, they urged, would our neighbours say
if they saw wine being brought into our quarters ?
They themselves were strictly forbidden to touch it ;
yet it was proposed that Christians should be allowed
to swill down as much of it as they liked and diffuse
its odour far and wide and pollute the whole city ;
nay more, Mussulmans who visited me came away
belching forth fumes of wine. These pleas very
nearly ruined our case ; finally, however, the opinion
prevailed of those Pashas who used their authority on
our behalf and urged that the change of diet would
be unendurable and would inevitably cause disease
and death to many of our number. We were, therefore, allowed to choose one night on which we might
have as much wine as we wanted put ashore at the
sea-gate, which we regarded as the most convenient
spot. On the appointed night we were to have carts
and horses ready to convey the wine with the least
possible noise to the house. In this manner we retained our rights.

There were some Greeks who attempted to shake
the Sultan's resolve by the following stratagem.
Learning that he was to pass through some districts
which were thickly planted with vineyards, they

assembled in large numbers and rooted up the vines, and either heaped them in the road or loaded them on carts. When the Sultan reached the spot, wondering what was happening, he stopped and, calling the nearest of the men to him, asked them what they were doing. They replied that, since his proclamation forbade them to drink wine, they were pulling up the vines, for which they had no further use, in order to use them for firewood. To this Soleiman replied : ' You are doing wrong and have misunderstood my intention. I enjoined abstinence from wine, but I do not therefore prohibit the eating of grapes, which should be regarded as among the noblest fruits which God has bestowed upon the human race. There is no reason why you should not enjoy their fresh juice, so long as you do not store it in casks and pervert its proper use by your pernicious inventions. Do you consider that apple trees ought to be rooted up because they do not produce wine ? Cease, fools, and spare the vines which will yield you excellent fruit.' Thus the contrivance of the Greeks brought no result.

I now return to the plague which I have mentioned as having broken out under my roof. Wishing to escape it, I sent and asked Roostem if I might have his permission to remove to other quarters, where I might not be exposed to the risk of infection. Knowing his character I had some hesitation about taking this step, and only did so lest I should be thought neglectful of my own health and that of my people. Roostem answered that he would refer the matter to the Sultan, and the next day brought the following reply from his master : ' What did I mean and whither did I think of flying ? Did I not know that pestilence

is God's arrow, which does not miss its appointed
mark ?   Where could I hide so as to be outside its
range ?   If He wished me to be smitten, no flight or
hiding-place could avail me ; it was useless to avoid
inevitable fate.   His own house at the moment was
not free from plague ; yet he remained there.   I likewise should do better to remain where I was.'   Thus
I was obliged to remain in that plague-stricken house
of death.

It so happened that not long afterwards Roostem
was attacked by dropsy and died.   His successor was
Ali, the second of the Vizieral Pashas, a kind and
intelligent Turk if ever there was one.   When I sent
him my congratulations on his new dignity and the
gift of a fine silken robe, I received a courteous reply,
in which he bade me regard him as a friend on every
occasion and not be afraid to address myself to him
when I needed anything.   His acts fully accorded with
his promises.   My first experience of this occurred
when, after an interval, the plague again disturbed
my household and, after attacking several others,
carried off the man on whose help and support, under
God, we most depended for the preservation of our
health.   I thereupon sent to Ali and made the same
request as I had formerly addressed to Roostem.   He
replied that I had his permission to go where I pleased,
but that I should be wise to apply to the Sultan as
well, for fear lest he might come upon my men wandering about too freely and be angry at their leaving my
lodgings without his knowledge.   Much depended, he
said, upon the way in which any proposal was put
before the Sultan, and he would take care to present
the matter to him in such a manner that I had no need

to doubt about his consent. Shortly afterwards he informed me that I might go wherever I liked.

The most convenient retreat seemed to be the Island of Prinkipo (*n*), four hours' sail from the city and the pleasantest of the numerous little islands which lie near Constantinople, and containing two villages, whereas the others have only one or none at all.

I have said that death robbed us of the man on whom we used most to rely. This man was our doctor, William [Quacquelben], the worthy and faithful companion of my long exile. I had ransomed a man, who, without my knowing it, was, as it turned out, suffering from the plague. While William was trying to cure him, he failed to take proper precautions, and became himself infected with the fatal poison. He held the heretical opinion that, when the plague was abroad, there was more panic than actual danger, and that at such times the usual diseases of various kind occurred, but that, through panic, most of them were ascribed to the plague, and so any ulcer or boil was treated as a plague-spot. Thus, although he was sickening for plague, he was far from suspecting the truth, until the disease, which had been increased by his concealment, burst forth with such violence that he almost died in the arms of those who rushed to his help. Even then he could not be brought to believe that he was suffering from plague. When, on the very day before his death, I had sent to inquire how he felt, he replied that he was better, and asked me, if it was convenient, to come and see him. I sat with him for a long time while he told me how seriously ill he had been ; his senses, he said, and especially his eyesight, had been so weakened that he could not recognize any one ; this affection, however, had passed away and he had recovered the use of all his senses ; all that remained was a catarrh, which interfered with his respiration ; if this could be relieved, he would be quite well again immediately. As I left him, I remarked that I had been told that he had some kind of abscess on his chest. This he admitted, and throwing back the coverlet of the bed he showed it to me, declaring that it caused him no discomfort and was due to the knots on a doublet which he had put on for the first time and which was too tight. That evening, when, according to the regulations of my household, two of my servants had gone to attend him for the night and were preparing to put on him a clean shirt, he himself noticed on his body, when it was stripped, a purple spot, which they declared was a flea-bite. However, seeing more and larger spots, he exclaimed, ' These are no flea-bites, but a warning that death is at hand ; let us therefore act upon this warning.' He, therefore, spent all the night in prayer to God, in pious conversation, and in listening to the reading of the Bible ; then at dawn he passed away in the full assurance of divine mercy.

Thus I have lost a beloved friend and valuable supporter. The loss to the learned world is equally great. He had seen, learned, and noted many things which he intended some day to publish for the benefit of the public ; but death has prevented his well-laid schemes. So highly did I value his loyalty and experience that, if the crisis had passed and I had obtained permission to return, I should not have hesitated to leave him behind in Constantinople in my place. After his death my labours seemed to be doubled, and, now that I have returned without him, I feel that I have left part of my very self behind. Peace be upon the good man's spirit! I have set up a monument to him, on which I have borne well-deserved testimony to his virtues.

But to return to my island, where I spent three months with great satisfaction to myself. It was wonderfully quiet, quite free from crowds and noise. There were a few Greeks, with whom I found quarters ; but there was not a single Turk to spy upon my amusements by his continual presence, for the Turkish servants, to whom I had become quite accustomed, did not interfere with me. I was free to wander where I liked and to sail about among the numerous islands just as I pleased. There are abundant plants of various kinds, lavender, prickly myrtle, and burnet, and many others. The sea is full of numerous fish of every sort on which I used to try my wiles, sometimes with a hook, at other times with a net. Boats were obtainable with Greek fishermen, whom I employed to aid me.

I used to cross to some spot which gave hopes of pleasant surroundings and good sport. Sometimes it was my pleasure to indulge in open warfare and transfix with a three-pronged spear a crab or lobster as it scuttled along in the transparent shallows, and pull it into the boat ; but the pleasantest, as well as the most profitable, method was to fish with a seine or drag-net. A place having been chosen where the fishermen thought that there were plenty of fish, I had it surrounded by the drag-net in such a way that a large space was enclosed by the net itself and also by the long ropes by which the two ends of the net were dragged ashore. Round these ropes the sailors twisted numerous green boughs to frighten the fish

and prevent them from trying to escape and take
refuge in the deep water. Thus, when the two
extremities of the net were dragged ashore, the fish
were driven into a narrow space ; but, though alarmed,
they did not abandon themselves to their fate. Each
of them resorted to the devices which their instinct
had taught them. Some tried to escape from danger
by a bold leap over the net ; others buried themselves
in the sand, so as to avoid becoming entangled ; others
attempted to gnaw through the meshes, although they
were made of quite thick cord. These were chiefly
sea bream, a species which is armed with powerful
teeth. Their object is to bite through enough twine
to make a passage through which one of them can
escape, whereupon the whole shoal follows the leader,
so that not a single fish of all their number remains
for the fisherman. I was afraid of this (for I had been
warned) and stood in the bows with a pole in my hand,
with which I struck their jaws as they bit, much to the
amusement of my companions. I succeeded, however,
in preventing only a few of the many that were in the
net from making good their escape. Even a fish does
not lack cunning in the hour of danger. Plenty of
fish, however, of other kinds were caught—black-tails,
scorpion-fishes, weevers, wrasses, rock-fish, and sea-
perch. Their variety made them a pleasing sight, and
I enjoyed discovering their names and habits. At
nightfall I returned to camp with the bows of my
boat wreathed with laurels and loaded with spoil and
prisoners. Next day I shared the booty with Ali
Pasha and the master of his household, who declared
that the gift was most acceptable. . . .

When the weather prevented me from going on the

sea, I had to amuse myself by looking for plants which were rare or unfamiliar. Sometimes, for the sake of exercise, I would walk all round the island, taking with me a worthy monk of the Franciscan order, who, though quite young, was stout and un-accustomed to exert himself. He had come from a monastery at Pera to keep me company. Once when I was stepping out in order to warm myself, he had difficulty in keeping up with me, as he panted and snorted : ' What need,' he exclaimed, ' was there for such hurry ? Were we trying to escape or pursuing somebody ? Had we undertaken to carry letters of great importance, and had we hired ourselves out as couriers or dispatch-bearers ? ' Finally the sweat broke out through his garments and made a patch as large as a shield on his back. When we returned to our quarters, he filled the whole place with his groans and laments and hurled himself down on his bed, declaring that he was done for. ' Why,' he asked, ' should you be in a hurry to make away with one who had never done you any harm ? ' It was only with difficulty that, after frequent requests, he could be induced to come to the dinner-table.

From time to time friends from Constantinople and Pera visited me, and some Germans who belonged to Ali's household. When I asked them whether the plague was not abating, ' Most decidedly,' one of them replied. ' What, then, is the daily death-rate ? ' I asked. ' About five hundred.' ' Great Heavens ! ' I cried, ' and yet you say that the plague is abating ! How many deaths were there each day when it was at its worst ? ' ' As many as a thousand or twelve hundred,' he replied.

The Turks hold an opinion which makes them indifferent to, though not safe from, the plague. They are persuaded that the time and manner of each man's death is inscribed by God upon his forehead ; if, therefore, he is destined to die, it is useless for him to try to avert fate ; if he is not so destined, he is foolish to be afraid. And so they handle the garments and linen in which plague-stricken persons have died, even though they are still wet with the contagion of their sweat ; nay, they even wipe their faces with them. ' If,' they say, ' it is God's will that I should die, then die I must ; if not, it can do me no harm.' Thus contagion is spread far and wide, and sometimes whole families are exterminated.

While I was living in the islands I made the acquaintance of the Metropolitan Metrophanes, who was head of the monastery in Chalcis, one of the islands, a well-bred and learned man. He was anxious for the union of the Latin and Greek churches, and thus disagreed with the attitude adopted by most men of his race, who shun members of our Church as unclean and profane ; so convinced is each man that his own way of thought is the best.

When I had spent nearly two months in the island some of the Pashas began to be uneasy about my long absence, and spoke of the matter to Ali, saying that they thought it would be more convenient if I were recalled to the city. For what if I should try to escape ? They pointed out that I had ships ready at hand to secure my flight, and facilities of every kind, if I cared to use them. Ali told them not to be anxious, for he had no doubts of my good faith. However, he sent a cavasse to tell me of this. This man carried

out an inspection without making it obvious that he
was doing so, and finding nothing which indicated any
intention to escape on my part, he returned, after
receiving a present from me, with a message to Ali
that he need have no fear that I would do anything
to prejudice the confidence which he reposed in me.
So my stay in the country was prolonged into a third
month, and then I returned to the town at my own
good time, without being sent for.

From this period dates my close friendship with Ali
Pasha and our constant conversations about peace.
By origin a Dalmatian, he is the only really civilized
man whom I ever met among those Turkish barbarians. He is of a mild and calm disposition, polite,
highly intelligent ; he has a mind which can deal with
the most difficult problems, and a wide experience of
military and civil affairs. He is now well advanced in
years and has continually held high office. He is tall
of stature, and his face has a serious expression which
is full of charm. He is devoted to his master, and
nothing would please him better than to obtain for
him the peace and quiet which would enable him to
support in greater comfort his age and infirmities. He
is anxious to obtain by courtesy and fairness—in fact,
by treating me as a friend—the objects which Roostem
sought to gain by bullying and intimidation and threats.

Roostem was always gloomy and brutal, and wished
his words to be looked upon as orders. He knew
perfectly well what the political conditions and the
advanced years of the Sultan required, but he was
afraid that, if he showed any leniency in deed or word,
he might seem to have acted from motives of avarice,
for the Sultan strongly suspected him of taking bribes.

He, therefore, never deviated from his customary rudeness, in spite of his anxiety to patch up a peace. And so when any answer was given which did not please him he would not listen and brought the interview to an end, and I always left him apparently in a bad temper. I remember once I had been negotiating with him about terms of peace and he had rejected my proposals as unworthy of consideration, and had bidden me leave his presence if I had nothing better to offer : so I immediately got up and returned home, after just saying that I was not at liberty to make any suggestions for which I had not my master's sanction. As he imagined that I had spoken with more feeling than usual, he called back my interpreter and asked him whether I had been angry. When he denied this, Roostem went on : ' What is your opinion ? If I obtained from the Sultan the terms which Busbecq has several times suggested, do you think he would keep his word and give me the present which he has promised me ? ' The interpreter replied that he had no doubt about my scrupulously carrying out any promise I had made. ' Go home,' said Roostem, ' and ask him.' Now I had by me, ready for any emergency that might arise, the sum of 5,000 ducats in cash, which are the equivalent of 6,000 crowns. With this money I loaded my interpreter and bade him tell Roostem that here was a proof of my good faith and a first instalment ; the rest would follow when the business was completed (for I had promised a still larger sum). It was not, I said, my custom to break my word. Roostem was delighted to see the money, and handled it, and then returned it to the interpreter, saying, ' I do not doubt his good faith, but this busi-

ness is full of difficulties and I cannot make any
definite promise, nor do I yet know what my master's
attitude will be. Take the money back to the ambassador and ask him to keep it for me until I know how
matters are going to turn out. Meanwhile, let him
act as my banker.' This money, which I had counted
as spent, remained in my hands after all, for a few
months later death carried Roostem off.

I must now tell you of an act of kindness on the
part of the Emperor. Since it seemed no longer
necessary to retain this money, after first informing
him I used it for a year's expenses ; for our annual
expenditure amounted to this sum. I afterwards
regretted having done this, when I began to consider
how many years I had spent on my mission and in
what great toils and dangers I had been involved ;
1 felt, inasmuch as I knew the value of my services
and the generosity of my excellent master and his just
appreciation of the merits of his servants, that I had
missed an opportunity and omitted to ask for a sum
of money which had been unexpectedly saved, like
a lamb snatched from the jaws of a wolf. There were
many men at court who had received larger rewards
for far less valuable services. I resolved, therefore,
to remind the Emperor of these facts and to confess
my mistake and ask him to hand me back the whole
sum, and beg him, with his usual generosity, to
remedy a mistake which my carelessness had made
me commit. It was easy to make good my case before
so fair a judge ; he ordered the payment of 6,000
crowns from his treasury. If I ever allow myself to
forget so generous an act of kindness, I shall regard
myself as no longer worthy to live upon this earth.

But I must return from this digression to my subject —the different character and mentality of the two Pashas, Ali and Roostem. Ali, throughout his life, had been free from any suspicion of meanness, and was therefore never afraid that his courtesy or easiness of approach would incur the Sultan's blame. Roostem, on the other hand, was always avaricious and mean, and his first thoughts were always of his own interests and enrichment. My interviews with Roostem were always very brief; whereas Ali purposely extended them over several hours, and his kindliness made the time pass pleasantly. Meanwhile the Turks who had come to pay their respects or to consult him would fret and fume because my presence prevented the Pasha from giving them an audience. I myself used to suffer the pangs of hunger, for I was generally summoned to him after midday, and I almost always went without having taken a meal, in order that I might have as clear a brain as possible for conversation with a man of such keen intellect. At these conferences he always insisted that we should give our respective masters such advice as we each judged to accord most with their interests. 'He was well aware,' he said, ' that his own master, whose life was drawing to a close and who had had his fill of victories and glory, needed nothing so much as rest; at the same time (as I myself doubtless knew) peace and quiet were very much to my master's interest also. If he wished to promote the safety and tranquillity of his own people, he ought not to provoke the sleeping lion again to enter the arena. Just as looking-glasses are naturally empty but give back the reflection of any objects which may be placed before them, in like manner the minds of princes present as it were a clean surface to receive the impress of the ideas which are presented to them. We ought, therefore, to put before the minds of our masters those things which most conduce to their interests. We ought also to imitate good cooks, who do not season their dishes to suit the palate of this or that person, but consult the taste of all the guests ; so we, in determining the conditions of peace, ought so to arrange them that they may suit the wishes and susceptibilities of both parties.' He showed great skill in impressing these and similar doctrines upon me. Whenever circumstances allowed, he gave evidence of his kindly feeling towards me ; and if I, in my turn, showed myself ready to serve him, he received my advances with obvious gratitude.

It so happened about this time that, as he was returning home from the Divan and had come to a bend in the road where he usually bade farewell to his colleagues, he made his horse swerve too sharply and, being intent on his salutation, leaned forward with all his weight upon the horse's neck. The horse, which had not recovered its balance, could not support his weight and fell to the ground carrying its rider with it. When I heard of this I instructed my attendants to wait upon him and inquire whether the accident had had any ill effects. He was much pleased at this attention and, thanking me, replied that he was quite unhurt, adding that it was no wonder if a worn-out old soldier were liable to fall. Then, turning to those who were standing by, he said, ' It is impossible to do justice to the kindness which that Christian always displays towards me.'

He used sometimes to say that wealth and honour

and dignity had been abundantly showered upon him, but that now his sole desire was to serve his fellow men and so make his name live in the grateful memory of future ages.

We had been engaged for some time in negotiations about peace, and I was very sanguine of attaining the solution which I desired, when an incident occurred which might have endangered and upset everything.

A man of Greek birth, whom they honoured with the title of Despot, had made an inroad into Moldavia under the cover of the imperial troops which were guarding the Hungarian frontier and had occupied it, after driving out the Voivode who was holding the district. This greatly disturbed the Turks, who were afraid that the trouble, serious as it was in itself, might be only a beginning and might spread farther ; however, they thought it wise to hide their anxiety and not aggravate the situation by unseemly panic. But Ali thought that he ought not to let the matter pass without informing me and learning what was my opinion. It was made known to me by a member of his household that I was to be summoned in a few hours to discuss the question with him. This message, I must confess, seriously perturbed me. Our negotiations were almost complete, and we were like actors in a drama of which only one act still remains to be played. I was in great alarm lest this fresh incident should upset everything, and lest we should be like sailors who are swept out to sea again when in sight of port. As I had been warned, I was summoned to Ali Pasha, and he received me with his usual politeness. He discoursed about various subjects, chiefly concerned with the conclusion of peace, and there

was no hint in his countenance or words that any
change had taken place in the situation, until I was
preparing to depart and had risen to bid him farewell.
Then, as if the subject of Moldavia had only just
occurred to him, he asked me to resume my seat, and
said, just as one does when one remembers some
trifle, ' Of a truth, I almost forgot something which
I wished to say to you. Have you heard that your
Germans have marched into Moldavia ? ' ' Into
Moldavia ? ' I said, ' no, indeed ; and it seems to me
most improbable. What should the Germans be doing
in so distant a country as Moldavia ? ' ' But it is
quite true,' he replied, ' as you will find out for yourself.' And he began further to confirm his statement
and to assure me that reliable information had arrived.
' In fact,' he said, ' to put an end to your doubts, we
will arrange for the capture of a German whom we
can send to you, so that you may learn the truth from
him.' On this I took refuge in the statement that, in
any case, I was certain of one thing, that nothing had
been done by the Emperor's orders or on his instructions. I pointed out that the Germans were a free
nation and were accustomed to serve in foreign armies,
and that it was possible that some of them, after
fighting under the imperial generals, had enlisted
under some leader who needed mercenaries ; my own
opinion was that he would not be far wrong if he
attributed this disturbance to the Hungarian magnates
of that region, who, wearied by the wrongs which the
Turks heaped daily upon them, had determined to
pay them out. ' And, indeed,' I added, ' if I may say
what I think, I do not see that they can be blamed, if,
after having been so frequently provoked and hounded

on, they have remembered that they are men and have
made up their mind to exact vengeance. Is there
anything which your soldiers have not, for many years
past, regarded themselves as free to do in Hungary ?
What kind of outrage or hostile act against our citizens
have they failed to perpetrate ? *Here* hopes of peace
are held out, but *there* none of the ugliest aspects of
war are lacking. I myself have now been detained for
many years as a prisoner, and no one in my own
land knows with certainty whether I am alive or have
ceased to exist. Those who have borne your insults
so long deserve, in my opinion, not blame but praise,
if they seize the opportunity for revenge when it offers
itself.' ' So be it,' replied Ali, ' let them make the
best use of it they can, provided they keep within the
bounds of Hungary and the neighbourhood ; but that
they should actually invade Moldavia, which is only
a few days' journey from Adrianople, is quite intolerable.' To this I replied : ' You cannot expect men
who are more accustomed to handling arms than the
law to make nice and delicate distinctions. They
seized the first chance which presented itself and did
not think that they need consider in what direction
or how far they might proceed.' So I left him, and
he did not seem, as far as I could judge, at all angry ;
indeed, he did not show himself a whit less amenable
during the peace negotiations which we held on the
following days.

While we were engaged in these negotiations, I was
much touched by an act of kindness (for so I inter-
pret it), which I received from the ambassador of the
Most Christian King [of France]. There were in the
Sultan's prison at Constantinople thirteen persons,

most of them young men, including some German and some Dutch nobles who had come there by a remarkable accident. They had embarked at Venice on a ship which every year conveys to Syria, under the protection of the Venetian republic, those who wish to visit the Holy City of Jerusalem. Some of them had started from motives of piety, others from love of travel and visiting distant lands. Unfortunately for them, just at the time when they reached land, the forces of the Knights of Malta had made a descent upon that part of the coast of Phoenicia and laid it waste and had carried off numerous prisoners. The Syrians, whose parents, children, and relatives had been seized, since no other means was open to them of vengeance or of recovering the captives, laid hands upon these protégés of the Venetians and accused them of belonging to the pirates, and gave them the alternative of either securing the return of their relatives or else submitting to the same condition of servitude. It was in vain that they displayed the passports which they had received from the Venetian government or appealed to the law of nations and terms of treaties ; might prevailed over right, and they were carried off in chains to Constantinople. Their youth was greatly to their disadvantage ; for the Pashas refused to believe in the probability that motives of piety had made them journey to Jerusalem, because usually among the Turks none but men of advanced years undertake religious pilgrimages. When I heard of this, I left no stone unturned in my attempts to save them from their wretched condition ; but I achieved nothing. An appeal was made to the Venetian Baily (*n*), because the misfortune had occurred

while they were under the protection of that republic.
He could not deny that he ought to come to their aid,
but he protested that he could obtain no concessions
from such heartless savages as the Turks. Meanwhile,
I relieved their distress with every means of comfort
that lay in my power. Suddenly, one day quite unexpectedly, they all came to me and informed me that
they had been released, thanks to the ambassador of
the Most Christian King, whose efforts had secured
their release. I was greatly delighted at this unhoped-
for event, and took care that the ambassador should
receive my heartiest thanks. The ambassador, whose
name was Lavigne, as he was bidding farewell to
Soleiman on his departure and was kissing his hand
in accordance with the usual custom, had managed to
slip into it a petition, in which he requested that, as
a favour to his sovereign, these men, whose piety
had been the cause of their misfortune, should be
granted their liberty. Soleiman gave his consent and
ordered them to be released immediately. So I provided them with journey money and put them on board
ship and sent them to Venice and thence to their own
country.

This Lavigne had at first made himself unpleasant
to me in various ways. Whenever he could, he used
to thwart me in my negotiations, and did his best to
bring me into unmerited unpopularity with the Pashas.
He used to declare that, having been born in Belgium,
I was a subject of the King of Spain, and was as much
in the service of that king as in that of the Emperor.
He said that I gave the king information about everything that went on in Constantinople, and that I
had paid agents who told me all the closest secrets,

among whom Ibrahim, the First Dragoman of the Sultan, played the most important part. I will tell you more of this man later. All this occurred before peace had been concluded between the Kings of Spain and France ; when peace had been made, he seemed to seek an opportunity to make amends for his behaviour.

Lavigne used to express himself with a freedom of speech which was savage and brutal ; he was incapable of suppressing or hiding anything that came into his mind, however distasteful to his audience. The result was that even Roostem avoided intercourse with him, although other people shrank from conversation with Roostem on account of his bitter tongue. Lavigne used to send his interpreters to demand an interview ; Roostem resorted to evasion, and requested him to make known his wishes through the interpreters and so spare himself trouble, saying that the business could be transacted just as well without his presence. But all in vain, for he would immediately arrive and express such sentiments that Roostem could rarely listen to them without taking offence. On one occasion, for example, he was complaining that due consideration was not paid to his master. ' Perhaps you imagine,' he said, ' that Buda, Gran, Stuhlweissenburg, and the other Hungarian towns were captured by your valour. You are quite wrong ; it is all owing to us that you possess them ; for had there not been continual wars between our kings and those of Spain, so far from capturing them you would have hardly been safe from Charles V in Constantinople itself.' At this Roostem could restrain himself no longer, and bursting into a violent temper, exclaimed, ' Do you talk about your kings and those of Spain ? Why, my master is so mighty that, if all your Christian princes joined arms together and made war on him at once, he would not care a jot, but could easily defeat them all.' So saying he retired angrily into his chamber, after ordering the ambassador to go.

At this point I must not forget to tell you what I learned about a tribe which still inhabits the Crimea (n), and which, I had often been told, showed traces of German origin in speech and habits, and even in facial and bodily appearance. I had, therefore, long been anxious to see a member of this tribe and to procure, if possible, something written in that language. Hitherto, however, I had been unsuccessful. Chance at last to some extent satisfied my desires. Two delegates had been sent from that district to Constantinople to submit some kind of complaint to the Sultan in the name of the tribe. My interpreters happened to meet them, and, remembering what I had told them to do if such a chance occurred, brought them to dine at my house.

One of them was rather tall and had a certain ingenuous simplicity of expression, and might have passed for a Fleming or Batavian. The other was shorter and more thickly set and had a dark complexion ; he was a Greek by birth and language, but in the long course of trade had acquired a good knowledge of their language, whereas the first named, by residence among Greeks and long association with them, had acquired their language to the extent of forgetting his own.

When I asked him about the nature and habits of these people, he gave the sort of replies that I expected.

He said that the tribe was warlike and at the present day occupied numerous villages from which the Prince of the Tartars, when he required them, enrolled eight hundred musketeers, which formed the mainstay of his forces. Their chief towns were Mancup and Scivarin. He had much to say of the Tartars and their barbarous condition, though not a few men of remarkable intelligence were to be found among them, who could give brief and apposite answers to questions about serious matters. He quoted an apt saying of the Turks that other nations have their wisdom written down in books, but the Tartars have swallowed their books and keep their wisdom stored in their breasts and produce it as required, and talk as if they were divinely inspired. He said that they are very unclean in their habits ; if soup is placed upon the table, they do not ask for spoons but drink the liquid from the hollow of their hand. They slaughter horses and devour the flesh without cooking it, merely folding slices under the saddles of their horses and eating the meat when it is warm from the horse's heat with as much relish as if it had been daintily prepared. The chief of the tribe eats off a silver table. A horse's head is brought in for the first and last courses, just as with us butter has a place of honour at the beginning and end of a meal.

I will next write down a few of the many Germanic words which he repeated to me ; for there were just as many words which were quite different from ours, either from the nature of the language or else because his memory failed him and he gave foreign instead of native words. He prefixed the article *tho* or *the* before all the substantives. The following are the words

which were identical with or only a little different
from ours :

Broe, bread	*Tag*, day
Plut, blood	*Oeghene*, eyes
Stul, stool	*Bars*, beard
Hus, house	*Handa*, hand
Wingart, vine	*Boga*, bow
Reghen, rain	*Miera*, ant
Bruder, brother	*Rinck* or *Ringo*, ring
Schwester, sister	*Brunna*, fountain
Alt, old man	*Waghen*, wagon
Wintch, wind	*Apel*, apple
Silvir, silver	*Schieten*, to shoot (an
Goltz, gold	arrow)
Kor, corn	*Schlipen*, to sleep
Salt, salt	*Kommen*, to come
Fisct, fish	*Singhen*, to sing
Hoef, head	*Lachen*, to laugh
Thurn, door	*Criten*, to cry
Stern, star	*Geen*, to go
Sune, sun	*Breen*, to roast
Mine, moon	*Schwalch*, death

Knauen tag was ' good day ', *knauen* meaning
' good '. He also used numerous other words which
were not at all like our language, for example :

Iel, life, or health	*Rintch*, mountain
Ieltch, alive, or well	*Fers*, man
Iel uburt, may it be well	*Statz*, earth
Marzus, wedding	*Ada*, egg
Schuos, bride	*Ano*, hen
Baar, boy	*Telich*, foolish
Ael, stone	*Stap*, she-goat

Menus, flesh

Atochta, bad

Wichtgata, white

Mycha, sword

Lista, too little

Schedit, light

Borrotsch, wish

Cadariou, soldier

Gadeltha, beautiful

Kilemschkop, drink up a cupful

Tzo warthata, you have done

Ies varthata, he has done

Tch malthata, I say

When I asked him to count, he did so as follows : *Ita, tua, tria, fyder, fyuf, seis, sevene*, just as we Flemings do. For you men of Brabant, who make out that you talk German, always pride yourselves very much upon so doing and laugh at us for what you call our disgusting pronunciation of the word which you call *seven*. He then went on : *Athe, nyne, thiine, thiinita, thiinetua, thiinetria*, &c. Twenty he called *stega*, thirty *treithyen*, forty *furdeithien*, a hundred *sada*, a thousand *hazer*. He also repeated a song in this language which began like this :

> *Wara wara ingdolou :*
> *Seu te gira Galizu.*
> *Hæmisclep dorbiza ea. (n)*

I cannot decide whether these men are Goths or Saxons. If they are Saxons, I think they must have been brought there in the time of Charles the Great, who scattered that race over various regions of the earth ; there are, for example, cities in Transylvania still inhabited by Saxons. Possibly it was thought best that the most savage amongst them should be removed to a still greater distance and settled in the Crimea, where, though surrounded by enemies, they still retain their Christianity. If they are Goths, I am of opinion that they inhabited this district adjoining the Getae from an early period. One would not perhaps be far wrong in holding that the greater part of the stretch of territory between the island of Gothland and what is now called Perekop was once populated by Goths. It was from here that the different Gothic clans, the Visigoths and Ostrogoths, came, and from here that they carried their victorious arms all over the world ; this was the breeding-ground of their barbarian hordes.

So much for what I have learned about the Crimea from these men of Perekop. Next listen to the information which I obtained from a wandering Turk about the city and country of Cathay (China). He was a member of the sect which regards it as an act of piety to wander over distant lands and worship God on the highest mountains and in deserted and desolate places. He had traversed almost the whole of the East, where he said he had made acquaintance with Portuguese travellers ; then, kindled with a desire to visit the city and kingdom of Cathay, he had joined some merchants who were starting thither. These merchants assemble in large numbers and travel in a body to the confines of that realm. The journey is not possible, (n) or at any rate is very dangerous, for small bodies of men ; there are many tribes on the route who are treacherous towards travellers, and their attacks are to be feared every moment.

When they had journeyed a considerable distance beyond the territory of the Persians, they reached the cities of Samarkand, Bokhara, and Tashkend, and the other places which are inhabited by the successors of Tamerlane. Then followed great deserts and regions, inhabited some by fierce and inhospitable people, others by more civilized tribes ; but everywhere the lack of provisions and corn causes difficulties. Each traveller, therefore, provides himself with a stock of food and the necessities of life, which are loaded on a great number of camels. A large body of men travelling thus together is called a caravan. After many months of toil they reached the straits or barrier leading into the kingdom of Cathay ; for a great part of the dominion of the King of Cathay is inland and surrounded by rugged mountains and steep rocks, and can only be entered through a certain pass which is occupied by the King's garrisons. At this place they were asked what they brought with them, whence they came, and how many they were. Their answers were transmitted by the King's troops by means of smoke during the day and by fire during the night to the nearest beacon, which in its turn passed them on to the next beacon and so on, until, within a few hours, a message, which otherwise would take many days, reaches the King of Cathay and announces the arrival of the merchants. By the same method and with the same rapidity he transmits his reply, announcing what his pleasure is, whether all are to be admitted, or some excluded, or their departure delayed. Those who are admitted proceed under the charge of special guides, stopping at halting-places at suitable distances, where the necessary food and clothing are supplied at a reasonable price, until they reach Cathay itself. Here each has first to declare what he has brought with him, and then bestow upon the King, as a token of respect, whatever gift he deems suitable. It is also the custom that the King should be allowed to purchase at a fair valuation any goods which he likes. The rest they sell or barter by arrangement, a date for their return being fixed beforehand, until which time they are allowed to transact business and make bargains ; for the Cathayans do not sanction continued intercourse with foreigners, lest the national customs should be contaminated by any foreign taint. They are then conducted back, being entertained at the same places as on their outward journey.

The same pilgrim stated that the people of Cathay are very clever and are highly civilized and well governed ; they have a religion of their own which differs from Christianity, Judaism, and Mahomedanism, but is most closely akin to Judaism, apart from its ceremonies. The art of printing has been in use among them for many centuries past, as is proved by the printed books existing in the country. They use paper prepared from the cocoons of silkworms, and so thin that it can be printed on one side only, the other side being left blank. There are numerous shops in the city for the sale of a perfume which they call musk, and which is the blood of an animal of the size of a kid. No saleable article is so highly prized among them as the lion, an animal which is rare in those regions and much admired, and commands a high price.

These statements about the kingdom of Cathay I heard from the lips of this wanderer, and he must be responsible for them. Indeed, it is quite possible that, when I was questioning him about Cathay, he was really answering about some other neighbouring region, and that, in the words of the proverb, I was asking about a sickle and he was replying about a hoe. When he had finished his story, it occurred to me to

ask him whether he had brought back any rare root
or fruit or stone ? ' Nothing,' he replied, ' except
this little root, which I carry about for my own use ;
if I chew or swallow a very small piece of it when
I am faint or cold, I revive and become warm.' As
he said this, he gave it me to taste, warning me as he
did so that I ought to use it very sparingly. My
doctor, William [Quacquelben] (for it was before he
died), tasted it, and expressed his opinion, from the
heat with which it burnt his mouth, that it was true
aconite.

It naturally follows at this point that I should tell
you of the miracle worked by another Turkish wanderer
and monk. He used to go about in a tunic and white
cloak reaching to his feet and with long hair, much
as our painters depict the Apostles. But under this
respectable exterior was hidden the heart of an
impostor ; the Turks, however, respected him as
a famous worker of miracles. They also urged my
interpreters to take him to visit me ; so he dined with
me in a sober and modest manner. He then went
down into the court of the house and shortly afterwards returned carrying a stone of huge weight, with
which he struck his bare chest several blows which
would almost have felled an ox. Next he placed his
hand on a piece of iron which had been made white-
hot in a furnace lighted for the purpose ; he then put
it into his mouth and turned it round in every direction, making his saliva hiss. The piece of iron which
he put in his mouth was oblong, thicker and square
at one end, and so heated that it looked like a glowing
coal. Having done this, he replaced the iron in the
fire, and after saluting me and receiving a gift he

departed. My servants, who stood round, were lost in amazement, except one who thought himself cleverer than the others. ' You stupid people,' he said, ' why are you astonished at this ? Do you believe that these feats are real ? They are sleight-of-hand and optical illusions.' At the same time he seized the iron by the end which projected a long way from the furnace, intending to prove that it could be handled with impunity ; but no sooner had he seized it than he let go again, his palm and finger being so burnt that he took several days to recover. This incident was greeted with loud laughter from his companions, who kept asking him whether he believed now that it was hot or was still incredulous, and invited him to touch it again.

This same Turk related at dinner that the head of his monastery, a man famous for his sanctity and miracles, used to spread his cloak on the waters of a lake which was near the monastery and, sitting upon it, was gently borne along whithersoever he would. Another feat which he used to perform was that he was stripped and tied to a sheep, which had been skinned and prepared, in such a way that his arms were bound to its forefeet and his feet to its hindquarters, and was then thrown into a heated oven until the sheep was thoroughly roasted and fit to eat, and he himself gave orders that he should be taken out ; he then reappeared quite unhurt.

' I do not believe it,' you will say. No more do I ; I only tell you what I have heard ; but I can bear witness to the feat with the white-hot iron, which I saw with my own eyes. This, however, is not so extraordinary ; no doubt, while he was pretending to look for the stone in the courtyard, he had fortified his mouth with a medicine of some kind against the violence of the fire. That such medicaments have been discovered you are well aware. I remember once seeing a quack in the market-place at Venice handle molten lead and apparently wash his hands in it without suffering any hurt.

I have already related that a few days before Roostem's death the conditions of my captivity were relaxed. This was very welcome to me, because it enabled me to receive men of foreign and distant nationalities, from whom I learned much that amused me. Against this advantage, however, had to be set the inconvenience that my servants abused the facilities for freer exit, and would often wander about the city unescorted by Janissaries. Hence arose quarrels with the Turks and disturbances which greatly annoyed me. One example out of many will give you an idea of the sort of thing that happened continually.

Two of my servants had crossed over to Pera without the Janissaries, either because the latter were away from home or else because they thought that their company was unnecessary. One of them was my apothecary, the other my cellarer. Having finished the business for which they had gone to Pera, they had hired a boat in which to return to Constantinople. Scarcely had they taken their seats when a boy appeared from the judge, or Kadi, of the place, who bade them get out and give up the boat to his master. My men refused and pointed out that there were enough boats available in which the Kadi could cross, and that the boat in which they were had been hired by them. He insisted, however, and tried to turn them out by force. My men struggled and exerted all their efforts, and fisticuffs were exchanged. As all this took place within sight of the judge, who was now approaching, he could not restrain himself from rushing to the assistance of the boy, who was a favourite of his. But as he was hurrying heedlessly down the steps leading to the sea, which were slippery with ice (for it was winter), he missed his footing and would have pitched headlong into the sea—in fact his feet were actually wetted—if his companions had not come to his rescue. A cry was raised, and the Turks rushed together from the whole of Pera with shouts that Christians had laid violent hands upon the judge and had almost drowned him. They seized hold of my servants and with a great tumult haled them before the president, or judge who tries capital charges. Cudgels were being produced, and their feet were being fixed in the stocks, in which they might be held while they were bastinadoed in the usual manner. Meanwhile, one of my two servants, who was an Italian, in a state of furious anger, did not cease to cry out, ' *Vour chiopecklar vour :* strike, you dogs, strike. It is *we* who are the victims of injustice and have deserved no punishment. We are servants of the Imperial Ambassador ; you will be punished by the Sultan, when he learns of your behaviour.' All this, though not expressed in perfect Turkish, was, nevertheless, quite intelligible. One of the Turks in the crowd, who was amazed at his boldness, exclaimed : ' Do you think that this cock-eyed fellow ' (for he had lost one eye) ' is a human being ? Believe me, he is nothing of the kind ; he is one of those one-eyed evil spirits.' One of the voivodes, as they call their magistrates, who was struck with the man's presence of mind and anxious to do no more nor less than justice, came to the conclusion that it was best to send the men unharmed to Roostem. So off they went, accompanied by a huge crowd of false witnesses ready to overwhelm the innocent by their testimony. For the Turks regard it as an act of great piety to bear false witness against a Christian. They do not wait to be questioned but come of their own accord, as on this occasion. All with one voice, therefore, cried out that these brigands had dared to commit the atrocious crime of striking a judge with their fists ; indeed, if they had not been prevented, they would have drowned him. My men denied the charge and said that they were being undeservedly accused, and then disclosed the fact that they were my servants. Roostem quickly scented out that it was a case of malicious accusation ; in order, however, to conciliate the wrath of the excited populace, he put on a stern expression and announced that he would punish the prisoners himself, and quickly ordered them to be conducted to prison. Their imprisonment saved them from the violence of the angry crowd. Roostem heard the evidence of those witnesses whom he regarded as worthy of credit, and found that my men were innocent and that it was the judge who was to blame.

Through the interpreters I asked that my servants should be given back to me. Roostem regarded the matter as sufficiently important to be referred to the council ; for he was afraid, he said, that if the Sultan heard of it he would suspect that the injury done to the judge had been overlooked through the influence of money. I was at this time already on terms of some intimacy with Ali Pasha ; to him, therefore, I

complained, again through my interpreters, and demanded that an end should be put to the wrongs done
to my servants. Ali took up the case and bade me have no
fears, for the annoyance should quickly cease. Roostem,
however, did not hurry himself, being still afraid lest he
should seem to have favoured me in return for a bribe ;
and so he would rather have had the matter settled
in such a way that the judge should be left with no
ground of complaint. He announced that he thought
that the best course would be that I should conciliate
the judge with a sop of several pieces of gold, sug-
gesting that twenty-five ducats would suffice.   I
thanked him for his advice and told him that, if he
bade me throw forty ducats into the sea as a personal
favour to himself, I should not hesitate to do so ; but
in this affair it was a question not of money but of
principle. For if once the principle were established
that any one who had wronged my servants should
actually receive money for doing so, my resources
would never suffice. Any one whose garment was
beginning to become thin or torn would make up his
mind to attack my servants, knowing that he would
be paid for so doing and that he would receive money
from me to buy a new one. I protested that nothing
could be more undignified or more contrary to my
interests. The result was that my servants were sent
back to me, chiefly through the good offices of Ali
Pasha. The Venetian Baily, when he heard about it,
sent for one of my interpreters and begged him to tell
him how much I had spent over settling this quarrel,
and was informed that I had not spent a penny : to
this the Baily replied, ' If it had been we who were
involved, I can swear that we should have scarcely

got off with a payment of 200 ducats.' The man who came off worst was the worthy judge, who was removed from his post, because the Turks are accustomed to regard it as disgraceful and shameful for a Turk to be beaten by a Christian, as he had admitted having been beaten.

You ask for information about the Spanish commanders, who, you say, according to a rumour which has reached you, are stated to have been liberated from prison through me. They were de Sandé, who commanded the land forces, and the admirals of the Neapolitan and Sicilian fleets, Leyva and Requesens. I will tell you briefly how I managed the affair.

The conclusion of peace between the Kings of Spain and France (n) caused the Turks considerable annoyance, as far from suiting their interests, particularly when they discovered that the terms were quite other than they had believed at first. They had been quite sure that their name would appear at the head of the list of those who were to enjoy the advantages of this peace ; and so, when they were passed over, considering that they had been ungratefully treated, they hid their disappointment but sought an opportunity to show that their feelings were less cordial. Soleiman had written to the King of France to the effect that he approved of the peace, but reminding him that old friends do not easily become enemies, or old enemies friends. The displeasure caused to the Turks by this peace was of no little assistance to my negotiations, and I was further aided by Ali Pasha's goodwill to me and by Ibrahim's strong desire to show his gratitude towards me.

You remember that I mentioned above that, when

Lavigne was finding fault with me, he used at the same time to accuse Ibrahim on the ground that all the Turkish plans were betrayed by him to me. This Ibrahim was the Sultan's first dragoman, as they call an interpreter, and by birth a Pole. Lavigne hated him all the more because, in a deadly quarrel which he had had with his predecessor in the French embassy, de Codignac, he thought that Ibrahim had favoured his rival. It is a long story and has not much to do with the matter before us. Lavigne never forgot this, and was always bitterly opposed to Ibrahim, and whenever opportunity offered of conversing with the Pashas, every third word of his was used to attack him, and this went on until Ibrahim was deprived of his office and dismissed from public life.

The matter touched me very little, for I had never felt any friendliness for Ibrahim, but on the contrary a certain enmity, because I had often found him opposed to our cause. I was grieved, however, that a rumour should be spread that it was owing to me that he had been dismissed from office. While Ibrahim was thus living in a private station and visited by the sickness of mind which usually afflicts those who have ceased to occupy a former position of dignity, I sought by any service that was in my power to lighten his unhappy lot, and, when my negotiations about peace were at their busiest, I frequently employed him as an additional interpreter and used him as a means of communication with the Pashas. This Ali willingly tolerated both on account of his goodwill towards me and also because he knew that Ibrahim had been unjustly dismissed. Finally, I brought about his restoration to his former post of honour. This circumstance caused him to be closely attached to me, and his strongest desire was to prove himself mindful of and grateful for my services. Most devotedly did he everywhere plead my cause and never omitted any opportunity of winning for me any goodwill which he could command. The annoyance of the Turks at this newly concluded peace made his task all the easier. Owing to this feeling of irritation against the French, when a nobleman, Salviati, arrived in Constantinople to ask in the name of the Most Christian King that de Sandé should be liberated, he failed to obtain his request and his mission was fruitless. De Sandé had lived in great expectation that this embassy would be successful ; for he felt that, if it failed, all hope was over, and he had gone to great expense in buying presents with which to honour the Pashas and the Sultan himself in accordance with the custom. The departure of Salviati, to make a long story short, was the end of everything for him.

Alarmed at this, the servants whom de Sandé had employed as his intermediaries came to me and confessed that they had not the courage to inform him of a result which he so little expected ; all his hopes, they said, had centred on this embassy, and the disappointment would, they feared, be more than he could bear, and his despair would lead to illness, which in its turn would cause his death. They therefore begged me to come to their aid and myself write to him. I was for refusing, for I had neither the necessary arguments nor the eloquence to console a man so grievously afflicted. De Sandé was a man of great spirit and of a sanguine disposition and one who knew not fear. But men who are of such a temperament as to hope for whatever they desire, if they find everything going wrong or turning out contrary to their expectation, generally become so despondent that it is difficult to raise their spirits again to a state of equanimity.

While the negotiations were thus at a deadlock, the interpreter Ibrahim presented himself at an opportune moment, and when, in the course of our talk, mention had been made of the Spanish prisoners, he went so far as to state clearly that, if I demanded their release, my request would not be refused; he knew what he was saying and had good authority for his statement. He had previously thrown out rather vague hints with the object of making me believe that I could obtain their freedom if I exerted my influence, but he made little impression on my mind; for how could I venture to attempt such a thing while I was still uncertain of obtaining peace? I was further prevented by the fear that, if I asked at an inopportune time, I should not only myself effect nothing, but perhaps also hamper Salviati's negotiations. But when, after Salviati's departure, I saw that Ibrahim, a man who was closely attached to me, encouraged me to act, I thought that there must be something in what he said, and I began to listen to him, warning him, however, at the same time to be careful to what course he urged me and not to expose a friend to ridicule. This certainly would be the result if I unsuccessfully undertook a negotiation which was generally regarded as impracticable and had already met with a rebuff. Nevertheless, Ibrahim persisted and bade me have no misgivings; he would be responsible, and was convinced that I should be successful.

On the strength of Ibrahim's assurances I wrote to
de Sandé, and while informing him of the ill success
of Salviati's mission, bade him not despair, for, unless
the Turks were absolutely unreliable, there was every
ground for hope ; and I told him what I had learned
from Ibrahim. After these preliminaries, I consulted
some of my friends who had a wide experience of
Turkish life. They wished me every success, but confessed that they could not see how I could hope to
be successful in a request which had been recently
refused to the ambassador of a king who was an old
friend of the Sultan, especially as the question of peace
with the Empire was still unsettled ; they also pointed
out that past history showed how difficult it was to
obtain from the Turks the release of prisoners of note.
Nevertheless, I wrote to the Emperor telling him of
the hopes which I had formed, and begged him
earnestly to ask Soleiman to grant the prisoners their
liberty. To make a long story short, after generous
presents had been promised to the Pashas if they would
show themselves favourable and propitious to their
liberation, the prisoners were released from prison and
conducted to my quarters on the eve of the feast of
St. Lawrence.

De Sandé and Leyva could not have hated one
another more if they had been brothers ! It was,
therefore, necessary for a separate table to be provided for Leyva, with whom Requesens dined, while
de Sandé sat at the table with me. While we were
dining, the steward of the chargé d'affaires of the
French embassy arrived with some notes or other
which had come into his hands. De Sandé asked him
if he recognized him. ' I believe,' he replied, ' that

you are Don Alvaro.' ' Indeed I am,' said he, ' and will you please give your master my best compliments and tell him that you have seen me here a free man, thanks to the Ambassador here.' ' I can certainly see you,' he answered, ' but I can hardly believe my eyes.' De Sandé acted in this way because the *locum tenens* of the French ambassador, though in other respects a worthy man, was among those who could not be convinced that Soleiman would release the prisoners as a favour to the Emperor Ferdinand.

Before the prisoners were released, the Mufti, who is at the head of the Turkish religion, was first consulted as to whether it was lawful to exchange a few Christians for a larger number of Turks ; for I had promised that no fewer than forty Turkish captives— ordinary soldiers, it is true, and men of no position— should be given in exchange. The Mufti replied that two different authorities expressed different opinions, one approving and the other disapproving of the exchange. However, the more expedient alternative was adopted.

I have still to tell you of Bajazet's final disaster, for no doubt you expect me to tell you the story. I think you remember how he was thrown into prison by Sagthama [King of Persia]. From that time many messengers went to and fro from the Persian king to the Sultan, some even bearing the title of ambassador, with gifts of the usual kinds, such as tents of elaborate workmanship, Assyrian and Persian carpets, and a Koran, the book which contains their sacred mysteries. Animals of unusual kinds were also sent, among which I remember hearing that there was an Indian anteater, as large as a good-sized dog and very snappish and savage. The alleged reason of their coming was to effect a reconciliation between Bajazet and his father. Great honour was paid to them, and they were welcomed by the Pashas with sumptuous banquets.

In one of these feasts Ali desired that I should participate, and therefore sent me eight large china dishes full of sweetmeats. It was usual among the Romans to send food from their tables to their friends, and the custom has been retained to this day by the Spaniards. The Turks, however, are accustomed rather to carry off for themselves some dainty from a richly furnished feast ; but this is hardly ever done except by intimate friends and those who have wives and children at home. My guests used often to carry home from my table napkins full of dainty tit-bits, and were not afraid of soiling their silk robes with drops of gravy, although cleanliness is a matter of the greatest importance in their eyes. The mention of this recalls to my mind an amusing occurrence which I shall enjoy relating to you ; you will laugh at it, as I myself laughed at the time, and you must not despise laughter, which is man's particular privilege and the best cure for human misery. After all we are no Catos (*n*).

The Pashas are in the habit of giving a dinner to all who wish to come, no one being excluded, a few days before their fast, which corresponds to our Lent. Those who attend it are, however, almost all neighbours, clients, acquaintances, and friends. An oblong leather coverlet closely crowded with dishes is spread on the ground over a rug, and provides room for a large number of guests. The Pasha himself sits at the top of the table, with the men of higher rank round him ; then come the guests of lower station in a long line, until no more room remains. More stand behind (for the table will not hold them all at once), and when those who have obtained seats have satisfied their hunger, which does not take long (for they eat with great moderation and without talking), and have concluded their meal with a draught of water sweetened with honey or sugar, they salute their host and depart. Their places are then taken by some of those who stand waiting, who are succeeded by others, until soon a large number of guests have been fed at the same table, the servants meanwhile busily removing and washing the plates and dishes and supplying clean ones.

On one occasion a Pasha who was giving a feast of this kind in his house had invited a Sanjak-bey, who had chanced to come in, to sit next to him. In the next place to him but one was seated an old man of the class which they call Hodjas, that is, men of learning. The Hodja (*n*), seeing before him a large collection of different kinds of food, and having eaten his fill, wished to take something back for his wife, and began to look for his handkerchief but found that he had left it at home. He was not at a loss, however, and devised a plan of campaign on the spot. He laid hold of the head-dress which was hanging behind him (and belonged not to himself, as he thought, but to the Sanjak-bey) and packed it as full as he could, putting on the top a piece of bread to act as a cork and prevent anything from falling out ; for he had to put it back in its place for a moment, in order to bid his host farewell in the Turkish fashion, saluting his superiors by placing his hands on his breast or at his sides. Having performed his salutation he gathered up the head-dress, taking this time his own, and, as

he left the room, he carefully felt it and, to his astonishment, found that it was empty. However, he could
do nothing but wend his way sadly home.

Not long afterwards the Sanjak-bey also rose from
the table and, after doing obeisance to the Pasha, prepared to depart, in complete ignorance of the load
which was hanging behind him. However, at every
step the head-dress began to deliver itself of its contents, and the Sanjak-bey left a long trail of morsels
behind him. When every one laughed, he looked
behind him and saw to his shame that the head-
dress was disgorging fragments of food. The Pasha,
who guessed what had happened, called him back,
and bade him sit down again, and sent for the Hodja.
Then turning towards him he said, ' As you are a
neighbour and an old friend of mine, and have a wife
and children at home, and there was plenty for you
to take for them from my table, I am surprised that
you did not do so.' To this the Hodja replied, ' It is
not my fault, master, that I did not do so, but my
protecting genius must have been angry. Having
foolishly left my handkerchief at home, I had hidden
the remains of my meal in my head-dress, but when
I left the room I found that it had mysteriously become empty.' Thus the Sanjak-bey's blushes were
quenched, and the disappointment of the learned old
gentleman and the oddness of the incident gave the
bystanders more food for laughter.

But I must return to the subject of Bajazet. His
position was now desperate, since his hard-hearted
father was demanding that he should be delivered up
alive for punishment. The Persian king meanwhile
evaded the request and pretended to protect him, but

could not be relied upon. Soleiman at one moment used blandishments, reminding him of their treaty, under which he had agreed to have the same enemies and friends, while at another time he tried to frighten him by threats and menaces of war if Bajazet were not handed over. He had strengthened the garrisons of all the towns in his empire which were near the Persian frontier, and had poured troops into Mesopotamia and all along the Euphrates, chiefly from the imperial guard and the army which he has employed against Bajazet. Mehemet, the third Vizierial Pasha and Beyler-bey of Greece, was in command ; for Selim had already returned home. He also sent frequent messengers to the tribes known as the Georgians, who live between the Caspian and Black Seas and are neighbours of the Medes, urging them to take up arms against the Persians. They replied with considerable sagacity that they were not confident enough of their own strength to venture to attack Sagthama unaided, but that, if Soleiman arrived with an army and they saw him in person, they would know what action they ought to take and would lack neither counsel nor courage. The Hyrcanians, who lived still farther away and who are the surviving descendants of Tamerlane, were also invited to join in attacking the common enemy.

Soleiman wished it to be believed that he himself was about to go to Aleppo, a Syrian city on the banks of the Euphrates (n), as a base of operations against the Persian king. Indeed, the latter was considerably alarmed, having often experienced what war with Soleiman meant. But furious as the Sultan was, he was restrained by the opposition of his soldiers and their aversion from such a campaign ; they shrank from so unnatural a war and began to desert from the ranks. A good many of them, especially from among the cavalry, returned to Constantinople without arms, and were promptly bidden to go back ; they obeyed, but in such a spirit as to make it clear how they would behave if any accident or change in the situation occurred.

Thus when it had become pretty obvious to Soleiman that he could not make the Persian king hand over Bajazet alive—and he excused himself by saying that he feared the vengeance of his captive, if he should escape after such treatment—the Sultan came to the conclusion that the next best thing was that Bajazet should be executed in Persia. He hoped that he could effect this, because in his last letter the Persian king expressed his astonishment at the negligence which he had shown in so important a matter ; he had, he said, sent ambassadors to Constantinople on many occasions, but the Sultan had only sent letters and messengers—conduct which made him doubt whether he was really in earnest. ' Let him,' he wrote, ' depute noblemen of authority and reputation with whom he could negotiate and come to terms about this important business. The Sultan was under great obligations to him ; for the arrival of Bajazet had given him much trouble and he had incurred great expense before he had been able to seize him. All this ought to be taken into account.' Soleiman perceived from this that what he wanted was money, and so rather than involve himself in an unnecessary campaign, for which his age unfitted him, he resolved to follow the advice of the Pashas and employ money rather than arms against the King of Persia.

First of all he chose Hassan Aga, one of his chief chamberlains, to go as ambassador to Persia, and ordered that he should be accompanied by the Pasha of Marash, a venerable and distinguished personage. They were given full powers to act, and started in great haste in the middle of the winter. The journey proved very difficult, and they lost several members of their party, but they eventually reached the Persian court at Casbin.

They first asked permission to visit Bajazet, whom they found so disfigured with the filth and squalor of his prison and with his hair and beard so long that they did not know him until he had been shaved. It was only then that Hassan, who had been brought up with him from his earliest boyhood—and this was the chief reason why Soleiman had sent him on this mission—was able to recognize his features.

An agreement was made that the King of Persia should be compensated for the losses which he professed to have sustained, and should receive also a present which accorded with the importance of the occasion, and that then Soleiman should be allowed to put Bajazet to death. Hassan hastened back and reported to the Sultan the result of his mission. The present and the sum of money demanded were prepared and conveyed to the Persian frontier in charge of a Turkish escort. Hassan also returned, having been appointed executioner of the unhappy Bajazet, with orders from the Sultan to put him to death with his own hands. The bowstring was, therefore, put round Bajazet's neck, and he was strangled. He is said to have made a single request before he died, that he should be allowed to see his children and embrace

them for the last time, but all in vain. He was told
that ' he had better attend to the business in hand '.
Such was the outcome of Bajazet's ill-starred projects,
his end being hastened by the efforts which he made
to escape it. The same fate overtook his four sons.

One of Bajazet's sons, who was still an infant, had
been left behind at Amasia when he escaped, and had
been sent by his grandfather to Broussa and was
being brought up there. Soleiman, when he knew that
Bajazet was dead, sent a eunuch whom he could trust
to Broussa to put the child to death. The eunuch,
having a tender heart, had taken with him one of the
janitors, a man callous enough to commit any crime,
that he might carry out the execution. When the
janitor entered the room and was fitting the noose
round the child's neck, the child smiled at him and
lifted himself up as far as he could and tried to throw
his arms round his neck and kiss him. Brutal though
the man was, he was so touched that he could not bear
to do the deed, and fell fainting to the ground. The
eunuch, who was waiting outside the door, wondering
why he was so long, pushed his way in and found
the janitor stretched senseless on the floor. As he
could not leave his task unaccomplished, with his own
hand he crushed out the feeble life of the innocent
boy. . . .

When the news of Bajazet's death reached Constantinople, misgivings seized me about the success of
our negotiations. Our position indeed was excellent
and the desired result seemed to be in sight ; but
Bajazet's misfortune reawakened our anxiety lest the
Turks should again become overbearing and undo
what had been accomplished and return to less favour-

able terms. We had successfully steered past numerous rocks, including the defeat at Jerba, the imprisonment of Bajazet, and the unfortunate incident of the Voivode's expulsion from Moldavia ; two difficulties, however, still remained : Bajazet's death, as I have already said, and another to which I will refer presently.

Ali had been the first to inform me about the news through a slave of his household and in the following terms : ' I would have you know that Bajazet is no longer alive. You can no longer trifle with us relying on any help that he can give you. Remember that it is easier to renew an ancient friendship between two sovereigns who have the same religion than to establish a new alliance between princes of different faiths. Be sure of this, that it is not safe for you to try any further evasions and to raise difficulties where none exist.'

This message disturbed me very much, and as I had reasons to suspect its authenticity, I sent round to my friends and inquired whether really reliable information of Bajazet's death had arrived. They all replied that there was no longer any room for doubt. I understood, therefore, that I must draw in my sails ; I could no longer hope for better terms, and must be satisfied if I could hold the ground that I had won and maintain the terms already granted. The Sultan had had them before him for some time and had shown himself favourable to them, subject to a few additions and omissions, some of which, however, I regretted. A few points were still obscure and might give rise to controversy if they were interpreted in a malignant spirit. I used every effort that they might either be expunged, or else emended in a manner advantageous to our cause. The terms had already been submitted more than once to the Emperor, and he had expressed his gracious approval ; but I was not myself entirely satisfied, and was always anxious to add little points which would further our interests.

It was while I was engaged on these negotiations that, as I have already said, the news of Bajazet's death arrived. But before this a serious hitch had been caused by the defection of certain Hungarian nobles from the Voivode of Transylvania to the Emperor, or, to describe their action more accurately, their return from error to the path of duty. They brought over with them to the Emperor the fortresses and cities which they held.

This new turn of events was likely to disturb and upset all the negotiations for peace which were on foot. Indeed, it supplied the Turks with a plausible argument. They could urge that no change ought to have been made while the negotiations were in progress ; if we really wished for peace we ought to make full reparation for this wanton act ; we might do as we liked with the deserters, but the territory which they held ought to remain in the hands of the Voivode, who was a Turkish dependent and a privileged official. But not only did Ali make no proposal to this effect, but he readily approved the condition, which I had expressly included in the terms of peace, that the *status quo* should be maintained. The ambassadors, however, who had recently arrived from the Voivode did their best to keep the wound open and filled the court with their clamour, protesting that their unhappy young master was being betrayed, that the rights of friendship were being trampled under foot, and that enemies were being preferred to old friends. This outcry made an impression on all the other Pashas, but not on Ali. Eventually the terms of peace, which had already been settled, were adhered to.

Although I could have no doubts about my master's wishes, yet, mindful that in the entourage of a prince there are never lacking persons ready to blacken the services of others, however distinguished, especially if they be foreigners, I resolved that, as far as was practicable, everything should be reserved as free as possible for his decision. And so in my negotiations with Ali I managed to point out that, although the proposed conditions did not entirely conform with the Emperor's expectations, yet I was sure that he would accept them, provided that some one were sent with me who could explain anything in them which was obscure or could in any other way give rise to discussion. I suggested that for this purpose Ibrahim would be the most suitable person, since it was through him that the Pashas themselves knew how anxious the Emperor was for peace. He was easily induced to accept this proposal, and so the finishing touch was put to our long negotiations.

It is customary for the Pashas to invite an ambassador, who leaves Constantinople in good odour, to dinner in the Divan. But since I wished that everything should seem to be in suspense and undecided until a reply was brought from my master, this honour was not paid me, a loss which I bore with equanimity.

It was my wish to take back with me some fine horses, and so I instructed my servants to attend the market frequently in hopes of finding what I required. Hearing of this, Ali himself had a splendid thoroughbred of his own exposed in the market as though for sale.

My men hurried to the spot and bid for it, and, when 120 ducats was asked, offered eighty, not knowing who the owner was ; but the men in charge of the horse would not sell it at that price. A day or two afterwards, the same horse, with two others equally well bred, was sent me by Ali Pasha as a gift. One of them was a beautiful Arab riding horse. When I thanked him for his gift, the Pasha asked whether I did not think that the horse, which my men had wished to buy in the market for 80 ducats, was worth a good deal more. ' Much more,' I replied, ' but they had been instructed by me not to exceed that price, for fear lest I might lose heavily (as sometimes happens) by their purchasing, without knowing it, a horse which had hidden defects.' He then advised me about the feeding of Turkish horses at the beginning of a journey, namely, that they ought to be kept on small rations at first, and that I ought to travel by short stages until they had become accustomed to the work ; and he recommended me to spread the journey to Adrianople over nine or ten days instead of the usual five. He also gave me a really beautiful robe interwoven with gold and a box full of antidote to poison of the finest quality from Alexandria, and lastly a glass vessel full of balm, which he praised very highly. ' The other gifts which he had given me he did not,' he said, ' value very greatly, because they could be bought with money, but this was a rare present, than which his master could give nothing more precious to a friendly or allied prince. He had been Governor of Egypt for some years, and so had had the opportunity of acquiring it.' Two kinds of juice are produced from this plant : one is extracted from the oil of the leaves, which are boiled down, and is black and cheap ; the other, which is yellow, is distilled from an incision in the bark, and is the genuine article, some of which he presented to me.

He expressed a wish for certain gifts from me in return : a coat of mail of a size to fit his tall and stout frame, a sturdy charger to which he could trust himself without fear of a fall (for he has difficulty in finding a horse which is equal to his great weight), and, lastly, some bird's-eye maple, or similar wood, such as we use for inlaying tables.

From Soleiman I received nothing beyond the customary gifts which are presented to departing ambassadors, such as I had generally received on bidding him farewell on previous occasions. He briefly inveighed against the insolence of the Heydons (*n*) and the garrison at Szigeth. ' What,' he said, ' has been the good of having made peace here, if they are going to disturb it and continue to fight ? ' I told him that I would report his complaint to the Emperor, and that I hoped that the matter would be arranged.

Thus under favourable auspices I started on my long-desired journey towards the end of August [1562], taking back as the result of my eight years' mission a truce for eight years, which, unless any important change occurred, was easily capable of extension for as long a period as we wished.

On our arrival at Sofia, from which town, besides the road to Belgrade, another route leads to Ragusa, whence it is only a few days' passage to Venice, Leyva and Requesens asked permission to take the road for Ragusa in order that they might shorten their journey to Italy and carry out as quickly as possible the promise which they had made to send gifts to the Pashas and to discharge the debts which they had incurred for various expenses at Constantinople. They offered to give me letters for the Emperor expressing their gratitude to him for their liberation, and saying that they would gladly have thanked him in person, if they had not been prevented by the obligations to which I have referred. I made no difficulty about complying with their request. The death of Requesens, at an advanced age, before he could reach Ragusa, made me all the more glad that I had consented ; I was glad that I had done him a favour, since a refusal might have been alleged as partly responsible for his illness.

De Sandé and I accomplished the remainder of our journey cheerfully enough without encountering any serious hindrances. De Sandé is a cheery fellow, of infinite jest, and quite ready, if need be, to forget his anxieties and make merry. Every day provided food for gaiety and joke. Sometimes it amused us to leave our carriages and try which of us could keep up walking the longest. In this I easily proved superior, being thin and unburdened by a load of corpulence, while my opponent was stout and impeded by his weight, beside being sluggish from the effects of his long imprisonment. When we came to a village it amused us to see Ibrahim, who was following us with great dignity on horseback with his Turkish escort, dash up to us and entreat us by all we held dearest to mount again into our carriages, and not to disgrace the party by allowing men of our high rank to be seen journeying on foot, which the Turks regard as highly undignified. His eloquence sometimes induced us to re-enter our carriages; but very often we laughed and took no notice.

I will now give you an example of de Sandé's many witticisms. When we left Constantinople, not only was the heat still oppressive, but I was in so low a condition from the recent hot weather that I could hardly eat at all, or at any rate was content with very little. De Sandé, on the other hand, being a lusty fellow and accustomed to eat enormous meals, which he always took with me (*n*), devoured his food rather than ate it, and encouraged me to follow his example and show myself a man and eat lustily. His exhortations produced no result until at the beginning of October we were approaching the Austrian frontier. Here, owing partly to the climate and partly to the season, refreshed by the cooler atmosphere, I began to feel better in health and so ate more liberally than I had done during the earlier part of the journey. De Sandé, noticing this, exclaimed that he was amply rewarded for his trouble and that the toil and training which he had lavished upon me had not been thrown away, since under his tuition and guidance I had learnt how to eat, after having reached my present age without acquiring the science or practice of that very necessary art. He might, he said, owe me as great a sum as I cared to name for having delivered him from a Turkish prison, but my debt to him for having taught me to eat was equally great ! Thus with many a jest we reached Tolna.

[At Tolna a quarrel occurred between de Sandé's Spanish doctor and a Janissary, which was eventually settled by the intervention of Ibrahim.]

On the next day we continued our journey towards Buda, the doctor being as active as ever in spite of his serious bruises. When we were already within sight

234 OGIER DE BUSBECQ IV

of Buda, some members of the Pasha's household came
out by his orders to meet us, accompanied by several
cavasses. The most remarkable members of the party
were some young men on horseback who were adorned
in the following extraordinary manner. On their
heads, which were shaved almost bare, they had made
a long incision in the flesh and had inserted feathers
of some kind or other in the wound : they were
dripping with blood, but they concealed their pain as
though they did not feel it, and behaved gaily and
cheerfully. Just in front of me there were several of
them on foot, one of whom was walking with his bare
arms crossed over one another, both of them pierced
above the elbow with the kind of knife which we call
a ' Prague Knife '. Another, who was naked to the
middle, had cut two slits in the flesh of his loins, one
above the other, and had inserted a cudgel in the slits,
so that it hung as from a girdle. Another man had
fixed a horseshoe on the top of his head by several nails ;
this must have been done some time before, as the
nails had so fastened on the flesh as to be immovable.

With this escort we entered Buda, and were ushered
into the presence of the Pasha, with whom I had
a lengthy conversation about the observance of the
truce, while de Sandé stood by. The extraordinary
band of young men who showed such contempt for
pain had taken their stand inside the threshold of
the court. Noticing that I glanced towards them the
Pasha asked me what I thought of them. ' I like them
very much,' I replied, ' but they treat their skin in
a manner in which I should not like to treat my
clothes, which I prefer to have whole.' The Pasha
laughed and then dismissed us.

On the next day we reached Gran, whence we proceeded to Komorn on the river Waag, the first fortress
in the possession of the Emperor. On both banks of
the river the garrison of the place with the naval
auxiliaries, whom they call Nassadistas, were waiting
for us. Before I crossed, de Sandé came up to me
and disclosed the anxiety which he had long kept
hidden and, embracing me, again thanked me for the
recovery of his liberty ; he confessed that he had
hitherto felt sure that the Turks could not possibly
be acting with good faith in the matter, and that he
had, therefore, been in perpetual fear that he might
have to go back to Constantinople and spend his old
age in prison. Now at last he recognized that the
liberty which he owed to my kindness was sure and
certain, and on this account he would be under great
obligation to me as long as his life lasted.

A few days later we reached Vienna. The Emperor
Ferdinand was at the moment attending the Imperial
Diet with his son Maximilian, whose inauguration as
King of the Romans was being celebrated. I sent
information to the Emperor of my return and of the
arrival of Ibrahim, and asked his pleasure about him ;
for he was urgently requesting to be taken to Frankfort.
At first the Emperor replied that he thought it better
that the Turks should await his return in Vienna, since
it would be hardly advisable that such bitter enemies
should be conducted through the heart of the Empire
all the way from Vienna to Frankfort. But this meant
a long delay and might give the Turks a handle for
suspicion of various kinds ; there was really no cause
for alarm in the journey of Ibrahim and his suite
through the most flourishing part of the Empire, nay,

it was actually desirable, in order that he might thus estimate its strength and size, and above all, that he should be witness at Frankfort of the unanimity with which the greatest princes of the Empire designated Maximilian as the successor of his imperial father. When I wrote to the Emperor setting forth these considerations, he consented that Ibrahim and his followers should be conducted to Frankfort. So we set out thither by Prague, Bamberg, and Wurzburg. Ibrahim was anxious not to pass through Bohemia without paying his respects to the Archduke Ferdinand. The Archduke, however, did not think fit to have an official meeting with him.

When I was within a few days' journey of Frankfort, I resolved to warn the Emperor about several matters connected with my embassy, and to arrive for this purpose a day or two ahead of the Turks. I therefore took post-horses and reached Frankfort on the eve of the date upon which several years before I had begun my second journey to Constantinople. My gracious Sovereign received me with a courtesy and indulgence which I was far from meriting, but which was in keeping with his usual custom and natural kindness of heart. You can picture my pleasure, after so many years of absence, at seeing my master not only in good health but also enjoying every kind of prosperity. He showed his satisfaction at the successful termination of my mission, which had fulfilled all his expectations, and expressed his gratitude and appreciation for my devoted services and the negotiations which I had carried out, and left nothing unsaid which could betoken his cordial goodwill.

On the eve of the inauguration Ibrahim reached

Frankfort quite late in the evening after the gates had
been shut, which, by ancient custom, are not allowed
to be opened during the whole of the following day.
But by a special order of his Imperial Majesty permission was given for them to be opened for the Turks
the next morning. A place was assigned to them
whence they could see the newly elected Emperor pass
by with all pomp and ceremony. They fully appre-
ciated what was truly a grand and splendid spectacle.
Amongst the rest who accompanied the Emperor in
a place of honour, the three Dukes of Saxony, Bavaria,
and Juliers (n) were pointed out to them, each of whom,
of his own resources, could have put a regular army
into the field ; and many other proofs of the strength,
dignity, and greatness of the Empire were presented
to their gaze.

A few days later Ibrahim was received in audience
by the Emperor and explained the reasons of his
arrival and presented such gifts as are held most
honourable by the Turks. After the peace had been
ratified, the Emperor bestowed splendid presents upon
him and sent him back to Soleiman.

I am anxious to escape from the court and return to
my own home, but private business still detains me here.
. . . In my eyes a life of retirement and peaceful study
is far preferable to the throng and clamour of a court.
But eager as I am to depart, I am afraid that my
gracious master may keep me here, or else send for
me when I have gone to the retirement of my home.
He has, it is true, assented to my departure, but only
on condition that I return if he sends for me. If
remain I must (and who can refuse the courteous
request of one who has power to command what he

will and to whom one owes so much ?) I shall be able
to find pleasure in the consolation that I can con-
template continually and gaze upon the countenance
of my revered Emperor, nay, upon the living image of
true virtue. For I assure you that the sun has never
shone upon a nobler prince or one more worthy to be
entrusted with the rule of an empire. Supreme power
must always win men's homage ; but for a monarch
to deserve such power and to prove himself worthy
of it seems to me something far more noble. . . .

There may, perhaps, be some who regret that the
Emperor has not shown more zeal for warlike achievements and has not sought laurels in that field. The
Turks, it may be urged, have raged over Hungary
for many years, laying it waste far and wide, and we
have never come to the rescue, as our reputation
demands ; we ought long ago to have marched against
them and, massing all our forces together, decided in
a pitched battle which nation fortune desired should
rule. Such advice is bold, but I doubt whether it is
wise. Let us consider the matter rather more closely.
In my opinion we ought to judge of the capacity of
generals and emperors rather by their plans than by
their fortune and the results which they achieve. In
their plans they ought to take reckoning of their opportunities, their own strength, and the nature and
resources of their enemy. If an ordinary enemy, well
known to us, and lacking the prestige of victory, were
to attack our territory, and our forces were equal to
his, it would, I fear, be imputed to cowardice if we
did not face him and check his advance in a pitched
battle. But if our enemy were a scourge sent against
us by the anger of Heaven (such as was Attila in the

olden time, Tamerlane within the recollection of our grandfathers, and such as the Ottoman Sultans are in our own days), to whom nothing is an obstacle, and before whose advance everything falls—to hurl oneself precipitately against such a foe with a small and hastily levied army would deserve, I am afraid, the imputation not merely of rashness but even of madness.

Soleiman stands before us with all the terror inspired by his own successes and those of his ancestors ; he overruns the plain of Hungary with 200,000 horsemen ; he threatens Austria ; he menaces the rest of Germany ; he brings in his train all the nations that dwell between here and the Persian frontier. He is at the head of an army equipped with the resources of many kingdoms ; of the three continents into which our hemisphere is divided, each contributes its share to achieve our destruction. Like a thunderbolt he smites, shatters, and destroys whatever stands in his way ; he is at the head of veteran troops and a highly trained army, which is accustomed to his leadership ; he spreads far and wide the terror of his name. He roars like a lion along our frontier, seeking to break through, now here, now there. Before now nations threatened by much less serious peril have often left their native land before the pressure of a powerful foe and sought homes elsewhere. There is little credit in remaining calm in the face of trifling dangers ; but not to be alarmed by the approach of such an enemy as ours, while kingdoms crash in ruin around us, seems to me (n) to betoken Herculean courage. Yet the heroic Ferdinand stands his ground with invincible spirit, never deserts his post, and refuses to retreat from the position which he holds. He would fain possess such resources that he could stake his all on the hazard of a battle at his own risk and without incurring the charge of madness ; but prudence tempers these generous impulses. He sees what ruin any failure in so mighty an enterprise would entail upon his own faithful subjects, nay, upon Christianity in general, and deems it wrong for an individual to harbour designs for his private gratification which can only be carried out by calamitous sacrifices on the part of the State. He reflects how unequal the struggle will be if 25,000 or 30,000 infantry, together with a small force of cavalry, join battle with 200,000 cavalry supported by veteran infantry. What he must expect from such a contest is clear to him from the precedents of the past—the disasters of Nicopolis and Varna, and the plains of Mohacs still white with the bones of slaughtered Christians (n). . . .

The Emperor Ferdinand's plan was the same as that of Fabius Maximus (n) ; after estimating his own and Soleiman's resources, he judged that the last thing which a good general ought to do was to tempt fortune and encounter the attack of so formidable an enemy in a pitched battle. He, therefore, resolved to throw all his energies into the other alternative, namely, to delay and check the tide of invasion by the construction of dykes and ramparts and every kind of fortification.

It is now about forty years since Soleiman captured Belgrade, slew King Louis, and reduced Hungary, and so secured the prospect of possessing himself not only of this province but also of territory farther north. In this hope he besieged Vienna ; then, renewing the war, he captured Güns and again threatened Vienna, but this time only at a distance.

But what has he achieved by his mighty array, his unlimited resources, his countless hosts ? He has with difficulty clung to the portion of Hungary which he had already captured. He who used to make an end of mighty kingdoms in a single campaign, has won, as the reward of his expeditions, some scarcely fortified citadels and unimportant towns and has paid dearly for the fragment which he has gradually torn away from the vast mass of Hungary. He has once looked upon Vienna, it is true, but it was for the first and last time.

It is said that Soleiman has set before himself the achievement of three ambitions : namely, to see the completion of his mosque (n), which is indeed a sumptuous and splendid structure ; to restore the ancient aqueducts and give Constantinople a proper water supply ; and to capture Vienna. His first two objects have been achieved ; in his third ambition he has been baulked—I hope, for ever.

[Busbecq then continues his panegyric of Ferdinand, and describes his public and private virtues.]

You ask about my Greek books, and say that you have heard that I have brought back a number of curiosities, including some rare animals. As to the latter there is nothing of great interest. I have brought back a very tame ichneumon, an animal notable for its hatred of and internecine warfare with the crocodile and asp. I had a remarkably handsome weasel of the species called sable, but I lost it on the journey. I also brought with me several very fine thoroughbred horses—it is the first time any one has done so—and six female camels. I have brought back hardly any plants or herbs, but I have some botanical drawings

which I am keeping for Mattioli ; I also sent him
a good many specimens many years ago. Carpets and
linen embroidered with Babylonian work, swords,
bows, horse-trappings, articles of leather, chiefly horse-
leather, finely worked, and other trifling examples of
Turkish workmanship and ingenuity—of these I have,
or to speak more accurately, I had an abundance.
For I have but little left ; in this vast assembly of
princes and princesses at Frankfort, I make many
presents of my own freewill to do them honour, while
I am ashamed to refuse the many requests which are
made to me by others. The rest of my gifts have,
I think, been well bestowed ; but there is one thing
of which I regret that I have been so lavish, namely,
the balm, on the genuineness of which the doctors
have thrown doubts, on the ground that it does not
seem to possess all the qualities which Pliny's description demands. It may be that it has been extracted
from very old plants, which have lost something of
their strength, or there may be some other cause ; of
this, however, I am certain, that it was produced from
the shrubs which grow in the gardens of Matarieh,
near Cairo. . . .

I also brought back a large miscellaneous collection
of coins, the best of which I intend to present to my
master. I have also whole wagon-loads, whole ship-
loads, of Greek manuscripts. There are, I believe,
no fewer than 240 volumes, which I have sent by sea
to Venice, whence they are to be conveyed to Vienna.
They are destined for the imperial library. Many of
them are quite ordinary, but some of them are not to
be despised. I hunted them out from all sorts of
corners, so as to make, as it were, a final gleaning of

all merchandise of this kind. One treasure I left behind in Constantinople, a manuscript of Dioscurides, extremely ancient and written in majuscules, with drawings of the plants and containing also, if I am not mistaken, some fragments of Cratevas and a small treatise on birds. It belongs to a Jew, the son of Hamon, who, while he was still alive, was physician to Soleiman. I should like to have bought it, but the price frightened me ; for a hundred ducats was named, a sum which would suit the Emperor's purse better than mine. I shall not cease to urge the Emperor to ransom so noble an author from such slavery (n). The manuscript, owing to its age, is in a bad state, being externally so worm-eaten that scarcely any one, if he saw it lying in the road, would bother to pick it up.

But enough of this letter ; you may expect me in person before long. Anything else I have to say shall be kept for our meeting. But take care to provide men of worth and learning to meet me, the pleasantness of whose conversation and company may enable me to rid myself of any traces of boredom and depression that still cling to me as the result of my long sojourn among the Turks. Farewell.

NOTES

PAGE 1. *1 Sept. 1555.* The date given in the Elzevir edition is 1554, which is impossible, since Busbecq only left Vienna for Constantinople in November 1554 after attending the marriage of Philip of Spain and Queen Mary in July 1554. It was on his return from his first mission to Turkey in the autumn of the following year that this letter was written.

The marriage of King Philip and Queen Mary : see Introduction, p. xi.

PAGE 3. *Gerard Velduvic.* He went as ambassador to Turkey in 1545.

PAGE 13. *Valpovat* : probably Vukovar, a small town dominated by a castle, on the right bank of the Danube about twenty miles south of the point where the Drave joins it.

PAGE 14. *King Louis* : see Introduction, p. xiii.

PAGE 15. *The place where there still remained traces of the piles of Trajan's Bridge.* As Busbecq followed the Morava from Semandria to Jagodina, he was at least eighty miles away from the site of Trajan's Bridge near Severin, not far from the point where the Danube issues from the Iron Gates.

PAGE 23. *Cantacuzeni and Palaeologi.* John Cantacuzenus, emperor and historian, ruled from 1341 to 1354 ; the name still survives in Roumania. The first member of the dynasty of the Palaeologi was Michael, who recovered Constantinople from the Latins in 1261. The last emperor of this family was Constantine XII, who was killed at the capture of Constantinople by the Turks in 1453.

Dionysius at Corinth. Dionysius II, tyrant of Syracuse, was deposed and banished, and became a schoolmaster at Corinth.

Baldwin the Elder, Count of Flanders. Baldwin I was elected emperor in 1204 during the occupation of Constantinople by the Latins after the Fourth Crusade. He died a prisoner in the following year.

PAGE 24. *Greece.* Busbecq uses Greece as a wide term covering all the country formerly occupied by Greeks.

PAGE 25. *Selim.* Selim I, who ruled from 1512 to 1520, was son of Bajazet II and father of Soleiman.

PAGE 26. *Two lovely arms of the sea* : the Bujuk Chekmeje and the Kuchuk Chekmeje.

PAGE 28. *Bajazet I* reigned from 1389 to 1402.

PAGE 29. *Tamerlane* (a corruption of Timour lenk, Timour the lame), the Mogul conqueror, after subduing Persia, Turkestan, Russia, and Hindostan, in 1400 declared war on Bajazet I. Invading Syria he sacked Aleppo and captured Damascus and Bagdad, and finally met and defeated Bajazet at the battle of Angora, 28 July 1402.

PAGE 36. *The people of Chalcedon . . . were called blind.* When the original colony was being sent out to Byzantium, the oracle advised that the new city should be founded ' opposite the city of the blind ', the people of Chalcedon having shown themselves blind in choosing the inferior site on the Asiatic coast opposite Constantinople.

PAGE 37. *Two serpents of bronze.* The serpent column, which consists of three, not two, serpents intertwined, still stands where Busbecq saw it in front of the mosque of the Sultan Achmed. Though Busbecq was unaware of the fact, it came originally from Delphi, where it supported the golden tripod set up by the victorious Greek states who defeated the Persians at the battle of Plataea, and whose names are inscribed upon it.

A fine obelisk. This was erected by the Emperor Theodosius and still stands on the site of the Hippodrome where Busbecq saw it.

This column is covered with reliefs. This monument, now destroyed, was also erected by Theodosius (not by Arcadius, as Busbecq states), and stood on the hill now occupied by the Turkish War Office. It was modelled upon the column of Marcus Aurelius at Rome.

The column which stands opposite the apartments, &c. This is the well-known ' Burnt Column ', which still stands in much the same condition as Busbecq describes. There is a tradition that when it falls the Turkish power in Europe will come to an end.

PAGE 39. *Corinth*. There was a proverb both in Greek and in Latin (quoted by Horace, *Epistles*, i. 17, 36) that ' not every one can go to Corinth '. This is interpreted by Busbecq as referring to the difficulty of entering the harbour of Corinth, but it was originally used, in all probability, of the expensiveness of the pleasures of that city.

The famous battle, &c. The battle of Tscaldiran (A. D. 1514).

PAGE 40. *Greece* : see note on Page 24, *Greece*.

PAGE 42. *a prison for distinguished captives*. In the Castle of Roumeli Hissar are still to be seen inscribed on the walls the names of unhappy prisoners, some of whom were ambassadors of European states.

The ' Clashing Rocks '. These rocks, which legend places at the entrance of the Black Sea, figure in the story of the Argonauts, who escaped destruction by sending a dove in front of them and then sailing through as the rocks opened again.

PAGE 43. *The burial-place of Hannibal*. Hannibal, after his defeat by the Romans at the battle of Zama (202 B. C.), fled first to Syria and then to the court of Prusias, King of Bithynia, where he took poison in 182 B. C.

PAGE 44. The *Ascanian Lake* : now the Lake of Isnik.

PAGE 45. *The Nicene Council* : the Oecumenical Council held at Nicaea in A. D. 325, at which the Nicene Creed was drawn up.

PAGE 46. *Chiausada* : perhaps Chakur Hissar.

PAGE 49. *the Sultana* : Roxalana, see p. 28.

Galatia. The province of Angora (now the capital of the Turkish Republic) occupies practically the same area as the ancient Galatia. The name of Galatia was derived from the survivors of the hordes of Gaulish invaders who were settled in that district after their defeat by Attalus, King of Pergamon, in 241 B. C. The ' Dying Gaul ' is a copy of one of the many monuments erected to commemorate their defeat.

PAGE 50. *a very fine inscription*. This is the *Monumentum Ancyranum*, the most famous of all Latin historical inscriptions. Its discovery and the recognition of its importance is one of the chief of Busbecq's claims to the gratitude of students of antiquity. The best English account of this monument is that of E. G. Hardy, *The Monumentum Ancyranum* (Oxford, 1922).

PAGE 51. *Balygazar, Zarekuct, and Zermec Zii.* None of these places can be identified.

PAGE 52. *Galen* : the famous medical writer of the second century after Christ.

PAGE 54. *a famous establishment of Turkish monks.* This is, no doubt, the Tekke or monastery of the Bektashi Dervishes which is mentioned by the traveller Evliya (*Travels*, trans. von Hammer, ii. 233) as situated near Tchoroum.

PAGE 59. *the Sultan Amurath.* Amurath, or Murad I, who reigned from 1360 to 1389, conquered the greater part of the European territory of the Eastern Empire and established his capital at Adrianople. He first instituted the Corps of Janissaries.

PAGE 67. *his zeal for the Persians.* The followers of Mahomet have from quite early times been divided into two main sects, the Sunnites and Shiites. The Sunnites accept the Sunna, or traditional part of the Law, and acknowledge the three immediate successors of the Prophets, the Caliphs Abubeker, Omar, and Othman. These tenets are held by the Ottoman Turks. The Shiites repudiate the Sunna and refuse to acknowledge the three successors of the Prophet. This doctrine had a zealous champion in Ismael, the founder of the Saffide Dynasty in Persia, and prevailed in that country, whence it spread to parts of the Ottoman Empire. It was rigorously suppressed by Selim, the father of Soleiman, who carried out a wholesale massacre of Shiites in 1513.

PAGE 69. *Lemnian earth.* This was highly prized for its medicinal qualities, being used, amongst other purposes, as a cure for dysentery, a salve for wounds, and an antidote for snake-bites. It was dug up with great solemnity on one day only in the year, the Feast of the Transfiguration (6 August) (see p. 136), and was made up into cakes on which characters were imprinted ; hence it is sometimes called *terra sigillata*. The name ' goat's seal ' often applied to it is derived from the fact that goat's blood was used in the mixture. All the evidence, both ancient and modern, about Lemnian earth has been collected by F. W. Hasluck (*Annual of the British School of Athens*, xvi (1909–10), pp. 71 ff.).

PAGE 71. *the defeat of Katzianer.* In 1537, in order to check the inroads of the Pasha of Bosnia into Hungary, a large force was sent under Katzianer, who was defeated near Essek. Katzianer afterwards entered into treasonable negotiations with the Turks and was murdered by one of his own countrymen. *Lasquen* is apparently to be identified with Lapancsa, which lies between Essek and Mohacs.

PAGE 72. *the defeat of Louis of Hungary.* See Introduction, p. xiii.

PAGE 74. *some sort of mushroom.* Agrippina is said to have poisoned the Emperor Claudius with a dish of mushrooms.

PAGE 75. *The line of Plautus.* The quotation is from Plautus, *Curculio*, I. i. 55.

PAGE 76. *14 July 1556.* The Elzevir edition gives the year as 1555, at which time Busbecq was on the journey in Asia Minor which he describes in the first letter.

Thrace. Busbecq uses the ancient name of Turkey in Europe.

PAGE 81. *Mahomet*, the eldest son of Soleiman and Roxolana ; see p. 79.

PAGE 83. *the inevitableness of fate.* The Elzevir text reads *facti*, which is a misprint for *fati*.

PAGE 84. *Facilis descensus Averni.* Vergil, *Aeneid*, vi. 126, where the received text reads *Averno*.

PAGE 86. *the Temple of Janus* at Rome was only closed in time of peace.

PAGE 98. *preparing to skirmish with a pygmy.* The legend of the battle between the cranes and the pygmies is as old as Homer (*Iliad*, iii. 2–6).

PAGE 115. *the Venetian Baily.* The Venetians and other Italian states, who controlled most of the trade in Turkey, enjoyed special privileges under Turkish rule as also they had done under the Byzantine emperors. In particular, they had a right of protection both of their persons and of their possessions under the jurisdiction of their ambassador, who bore the title of Baily. This system eventually developed into the so-called Capitulations, only abolished in 1914, which gave certain foreign powers the right to appoint their own magistrates to try their subjects in the Ottoman Empire.

PAGE 116. *Thus the man was saved.* This story is quoted
by Bacon in his thirteenth essay.

PAGE 121. *Turks and Persians* : see note on p. 67.

PAGE 130. *plenty of Medeas.* Medea, who fell in love with
Jason when he came to her land with the Argonauts, was
daughter of the King of Colchis, and therefore came from the
district inhabited by the Mingrelians.

   Godfrey de Bouillon. It is difficult to see how Godfrey
de Bouillon, who took part in the First Crusade and became
King of Jerusalem, could have introduced the story of Roland
to a tribe living in the Caucasus.

PAGE 134. *the Turks, like us, have an Easter.* The Feast
of Bairam resembles the Christian Easter in coming at the
end of Ramazan, the month of fast ; for which see pp. 151 ff.
For Bairam see pp. 161 ff.

PAGE 136. ' *Goat's Seal* ' : see note on p. 69, *Lemnian
earth.*

PAGE 155. ' *Give me another one.*' This is an allusion to
Tacitus, *Annals*, i. 23, where the words are applied to a
Roman centurion who was fond of flogging his men.

PAGE 163. *on the pretence of religion.* The Saffide dynasty
had been founded by Shah Ismael, the father of Sagthama,
who had established Shiism as the religion of Persia. See
note on p. 67, *his zeal for the Persians.*

PAGE 168. *a Greek land* : see note on p. 40, *Greece.*

PAGE 169. *Jerba.* This island lies off the coast of Tunis
in the Bay of Cabes. Towards the end of the year 1559 the
Duke of Medina, Viceroy of Sicily, set out with a fleet which
included contingents from several Italian states, in order to
make war on the corsairs who infested the Mediterranean.
He occupied Jerba as a base of operations. Busbecq's
account of the sudden arrival of the Turkish fleet, which
attacked the island and inflicted what was the most serious
defeat ever sustained by a Christian fleet at the hands of the
Turks, is a valuable authority on these events, since he no
doubt derived his information at first hand from the captives
who were brought to Constantinople.

PAGE 176. *Black Sea.* The Latin text reads *maris rubri*,
' Red Sea ', an error on the part of the author or his printer.

PAGE 184. *Prinkipo.* This is the largest of the Prince's

Islands in the Sea of Marmora some fourteen miles south-east of Constantinople. It is a favourite summer resort at the present day.

PAGE 198. *the Venetian Baily* : see note on p. 115.

PAGE 201. *a tribe which still inhabits the Crimea*. The data which Busbecq has collected about the Crim-Gothic language is invaluable from a philological point of view as the latest evidence we possess about the language. The continued existence of members of this branch of the Gothic people must have been due to their isolated position in the Crimean peninsula, into which the Huns failed to penetrate when they swept across southern Russia. Those who are interested in the subject may be referred to the following writers : Henry Bradley, *The Goths* (London, 1887), pp. 363 f. ; R. Loewe, *Die Reste der Germanen am Schwarzen Meere* (Halle, 1896) ; Tomaschek, *Die Goten in Taurien* (Vienna, 1881) ; F. Kluge, *Altgermanische Dialekte* (Strassburg, 1906), pp. 515 f. For the Gothic language in general reference may be made to Wright's *Gothic Grammar* (Oxford, 1910).

PAGE 204. *Wara wara ingdolou*, &c. While the eighty-six words contained in Busbecq's vocabulary are direct descendants of words found in Wulfila's Gothic Bible, these lines of verse are in a Turkish dialect (see Kum, *Codex Cumanicus*, p. 243).

PAGE 205. *The journey is not possible*. The sense here requires the insertion of a negative which is lacking in the Latin text.

PAGE 214. *peace between the Kings of Spain and France*. The reference is to the treaty of Cateau-Cambrésis (April 1559).

PAGE 220. *we are no Catos*. An allusion to Marcus Porcius Cato, the famous Roman censor.

PAGE 221. *The Hodja*. Busbecq does not seem to have been aware that the story which he tells here is one of a large number of traditional Turkish tales attributed to Nasreddin Hodja, the Turkish Joe Miller, an actual person who lived at Akshehir in the heart of Asia Minor in the fourteenth to fifteenth centuries. Some of the best of these stories are given by Sir William Whittall in an appendix to his book entitled *Frederick the Great on Kingcraft* (pp. 203–36) ; see also Sir Charles Eliot, *The Turks in Europe*, pp. 107 ff.

The following are two typical Hodja stories. On one occasion the Hodja killed a very fine hare and went about boasting of its great size. So the next day, when he was dining off broth made from the hare, four of his friends arrived, and with characteristic hospitality the Hodja asked them to partake of the broth ; but so large was the hare that the broth was not finished. So next day these friends sent four of *their* friends, who were likewise entertained, though on rather weaker broth. On the third day these sent four of *their* friends ; but by now the hare was finished, and all that could be set before the guests was some hot water in which the bones has been boiled. When the guests found fault with the Hodja for his lack of hospitality he said, ' Are you not the friends of the friends of the friends who dined off my hare ? ' And they replied, ' We are.' ' Even so,' said the Hodja, ' and what you are eating is the broth of the broth of the broth of that hare.'

On another occasion the Hodja woke up in the night and saw a thief dressed in white in his courtyard. So he put a shot through him and went back to bed. Next morning he went out early to bury the corpse and found that he had only shot a hole through his own shirt which was hanging out to dry. So he hurried to the nearest mosque and climbed the minaret and in a loud voice intoned a song of thanksgiving. The neighbours, annoyed at being roused so early, rushed out and remonstrated with him. ' My friends,' exclaimed the Hodja, ' would not *you* thank Allah for having saved *your* lives ? If I had been in that shirt, the shot would have passed through my heart and killed me.'

PAGE 223. *the Euphrates.* Aleppo is actually sixty miles from the nearest point on the Euphrates.

PAGE 231. *Heydons.* These were Hungarian irregulars : see p. 12.

PAGE 233. *which he always took with me. Mecum* must be read in the Latin text for *secum.*

PAGE 237. *the three Dukes of Saxony, Bavaria, and Juliers.* They were Augustus, Elector of Saxony, and Ferdinand's two sons-in-law, Albert III, Duke of Bavaria, and William,

Duke of Juliers, brother of Henry VIII's wife Anne of Cleves.

PAGE 239. *seems to me.* We must read *mihi* for *nihil* in the Latin text.

PAGE 240. *The disasters of Nicopolis,* &c. At the battle of Nicopolis (A. D. 1396) the Emperor Sigismond was defeated by the Sultan Bajazet I ; at Varna (A.D. 1444) Ladislaus, King of Hungary, was defeated by Murad II ; for Mohacs see Introduction, p. xiii.

Fabius Maximus. The Roman general who wore out Hannibal by marches and countermarches without coming to a regular engagement.

PAGE 241. *the completion of his mosque.* The mosque of the Sultan Soleiman is the most striking object on the sky-line as one looks across the Golden Horn from Pera to Stamboul. It was finished in 1555.

PAGE 243. *I shall not cease to urge the Emperor,* &c. It is gratifying to find that the Emperor purchased this manuscript, which is illustrated with remarkable miniatures and was the basis of Mattioli's great Editio Princeps of Dioscurides.

INDEX

EDWARD SEYMOUR FORSTER (1879-1950) was a lecturer in classics at the University of Sheffield from 1905 to 1945. He translated a number of Aristotle's works as well as other ancient texts for publication in the Loeb Classical Library series. He also wrote several books, including *A Short History of Modern Greece*. His translation of *Busbecq's Turkish Letters* first appeared in 1927.

KARL A. ROIDER is a professor of history at Louisiana State University and the author of four books, including *Austria's Eastern Question, 1700-1790*.